Essential Facts Geriatric Medicine

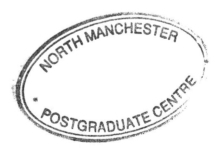

Catherine Bracewell
Consultant Physician in Geriatric Medicine and
General (Internal) Medicine
Newham University Hospital NHS Trust

Rosaire Gray
Consultant Physician in Geriatric Medicine,
General (Internal) Medicine and Cardiology
Whittington Hospital NHS Trust

Gurcharan S Rai
Consultant Physician in Geriatric Medicine
Whittington Hospital NHS Trust

Radcliffe Publishing
Oxford • Seattle

EQPAX

Radcliffe Publishing Ltd
18 Marcham Road
Abingdon
Oxon OX14 1AA
United Kingdom

www.radcliffe-oxford.com
Electronic catalogue and worldwide online ordering facility.

British Library Cataloguing in Publication Data

A catalogue record for this book is available from the British Library.

ISBN 978 1 85775 867 2

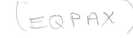

Typeset by Advance Typesetting Ltd, Oxford
Printed and bound by TJI Digital, Padstow, Cornwall

Contents

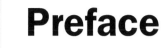

Preface

Demographic changes have led to an increasing number of older people presenting to family doctors and hospitals. The healthcare needs of these older people differ substantially from those of younger patients; older patients are more likely to have complex needs in view of the physical, psychological and social changes associated with ageing. In addition, presentation of illness may alter with ageing as may the response to treatment.

The Royal College of Physicians (RCP) has developed an examination for a Diploma in Geriatric Medicine. The aim is to assess the knowledge and competence of doctors providing care to older people in general practice, of clinicians with interest in or responsibilities for the care of older people, and of those working in departments of geriatric medicine in non-consultant grades.

Although this book is based on the syllabus for the written examination for the Diploma in Geriatric Medicine, it should prove valuable in every clinical practice and as a useful resource for junior doctors and medical students.

Catherine Bracewell
Rosaire Gray
Gurcharan S Rai
October 2004

About the authors

Dr Catherine Bracewell has just completed her training and is now practising as a Consultant Physician in Geriatric Medicine and General (Internal) Medicine at Newham University Hospital NHS Trust.

Dr Rosaire Gray is a Consultant Physician in Geriatric Medicine, General (Internal) Medicine and Cardiology at the Whittington Hospital NHS Trust. She is actively involved in teaching and training of junior medical staff and undergraduates and research. Her subspecialty areas of interest include stroke and syncope/falls.

Dr Gurcharan S Rai is a Consultant Physician in Geriatric Medicine at the Whittington Hospital. Since his appointment as Consultant Physician he has been actively involved in teaching and training of undergraduates and post-graduates, including those on general professional vocational training schemes, and at the present time he is chairman of the training committee in geriatric medicine in North Thames (East).

Abbreviations

AA	attendance allowance
ACTH	adrenocorticotrophic hormone
AD	Alzheimer's disease
ADL	activity of daily living
ACE-I	angiotensin-converting enzyme inhibitor
AF	atrial fibrillation
AMTS	abbreviated mental test score
APTT	activated partial thromboplastin time
bd	twice daily
BM	blood glucose measurement
BMA	British Medical Association
BMD	bone mineral density
BNP	B-type natriuretic peptide
BP	blood pressure
BPH	benign prostatic hypertrophy
BTS	British Thoracic Society
CA	carer's allowance
CAP	community-acquired pneumonia
CHD	coronary heart disease
COPD	chronic obstructive pulmonary disease
CPR	cardiopulmonary resuscitation
CSA	Care Standards Act
CSF	cerebrospinal fluid
CT	computed tomography
DBP	diastolic blood pressure
DC	direct current
DEXA	dual energy x-ray absorptiometry
DM	diabetes mellitus
DNAR	do not attempt resuscitation
DVLA	Driver and Vehicle Licensing Agency
ECG	electrocardiograph
ENT	ear, nose and throat
ESR	erythrocyte sedimentation rate
FBC	full blood count
FEV_1	forced expiratory volume in one second
FSH	follicle stimulating hormone
FVC	forced vital capacity
GFR	glomerular filtration rate

GH	growth hormone
GI	gastrointestinal
GMC	General Medical Council
HIV	human immunodeficiency virus
HONK	hyperosmolar nonketotic coma
HRT	hormone replacement therapy
ICP	intracranial pressure
IGF-1	insulin-like growth factor-1
IHD	ischaemic heart disease
INR	international normalised ratio
ISH	isolated systolic hypertension
kPa	kilopascals
LA	local authority
LACI	lacunar infarct
LBM	lean body mass
LFT	liver function test
LH	luteinising hormone
LTOT	long-term oxygen therapy
MCA	middle cerebral artery
MCS	microscopy, culture and sensitivity
MMSE	mini-mental state examination
MRI	magnetic resonance imaging
MRC	Medical Research Council
MIND	National Association for Mental Health
NICE	National Institute for Clinical Excellence
NMDA	N-methyl D-aspartate
NREM	non-rapid eye movement
NSAID	non-steroidal anti-inflammatory drug
NSF	National Service Framework
NTO	National Training Organisation
NVQ	National Vocational Qualification
OA	osteoarthritis
od	once daily
OCP	ova, cysts and parasites
PACI	partial anterior circulation infarction
POCI	posterior circulation infarction
PPI	proton pump inhibitor
PSA	prostate-specific antigen
PTH	parathyroid hormone
qds	four times a day
RCT	randomised controlled trial
REM	rapid eye movement
RNIB	Royal National Institute for the Blind
SaO2	oxygen saturations

SBP	systolic blood pressure
SSD	Social Services Department
T3	tri-iodothyronine
T4	thyroxine
TACI	total anterior circulation infarction
tds	three times a day
TENS	transcutaneous electrical nerve stimulation
TIA	transient ischaemic attack
TRH	thyrotropin releasing hormone
TSH	thyroid stimulating hormone
TURP	transurethral resection of the prostate
U+E	urea and electrolytes
UKCC	United Kingdom Care Commission
UKPDS	United Kingdom Prospective Diabetes Study
WHO	World Health Organization

Part I

Demographic and social factors

1

Demography of the ageing population of the United Kingdom

Background

- People are living longer.
- Birth rates are falling.
- A global shift in the age structure of populations is occurring with more people than ever aged over 65 years.
- This age shift has important health, social and economic consequences.
- Policies to enhance the health, independence and productivity of older people are vital.

Age structure of the population

- The population of the UK was 58 789 194 according to the 2001 Census.
- Of this total 18.4% were over pensionable age.
- Ethnic minority elders comprise approximately 7% of the population.
- Similar age shifts are occurring in other First World nations and in developing countries.
- The world's elderly population (over 65 years) is growing at a rate of 2.4% annually.
- In developed countries there are 165 million elderly people – this is expected to increase to 257 million by 2025.
- Sweden has the highest number of older people of the major countries of the world (17%) closely followed by the UK, Italy, Belgium and France (16%).
- The fastest growing segment of the elderly population is the 'old old' (over 80 years).

Future patterns of ageing

- Life expectancy is increasing with each generation: in 1999 it was 19.2 years for a man aged 60 and 22.8 years for a 60-year-old woman.
- By 2036 it is estimated that:
  - the number of 60–74 year olds will increase by 50%
  - the over-75 year age group will have increased by 70%
  - the 15–44 age group will have declined by 8%.
- The number of centenarians in England and Wales is increasing with time:
  - 1951: 300
  - 1996: 5523 (4943 women/580 men)
  - 2036: 39 000
  - 2066: 95 000.

Factors influencing ageing patterns and trends

- Low fertility rates (nearly all developed countries now have fertility rates below the natural replacement level of 2.1 children per woman).
- The postwar 'baby boom' will contribute to the accelerated growth of the older population in the second and third decades of the twenty-first century.
- Improving mortality rates.
- Increasing longevity.
- Medical treatment advances and improved health.
- Migration.

Implications of an ageing population on society

The age shift is far reaching in its implications.

Healthcare

- Disabilities and multiple health problems are more common in older people.

- Demands on the healthcare service will increase as the population ages.
- The World Health Organization (WHO) warns that the health impact of ageing could be enormous and predicts a large rise in cancer, ischaemic heart disease (IHD), diabetes mellitus (DM), dementia and other illnesses relating to old age.
- The elderly attend emergency departments more frequently than younger people.
- Inpatient length of stay is greater for the older person.
- GP home visits are most commonly to the elderly.

Social support

- A large proportion of home care services are dedicated to the elderly.
- A growing number of frail older people will necessitate the expansion of social service support for community dwellers and the number of places in residential and nursing care facilities.
- Smaller families, more women entering the workforce and younger family members migrating away from the home will mean that fewer people will be available to care for older people when they need assistance.

Economic consequences

More funding will be required, not just to augment health and social services, but to tackle other issues including employment, pensions, transport and town planning.

Planning for the age shift

- The challenges of population ageing are global, national and local.
- It is important to understand demographic trends to plan for the future.
- People without disabilities face fewer impediments to continued work, use less medical care and require fewer care-giving services.
- It is far less costly to prevent disease than to treat it.
- WHO has launched a campaign to promote good health in old age and has adopted the term 'active ageing: the process of optimising opportunities for physical, social and mental wellbeing throughout the life course, in order to extend healthy life expectancy, productivity and quality of life in older age'.

- The aims of 'active ageing' are to:
    - reduce the number of adults dying prematurely in the highly productive stages of life
    - reduce the number of disabilities associated with chronic diseases
    - ensure that older people remain independent and enjoy a positive quality of life
    - encourage older people to continue to make a productive contribution to the economy
    - reduce the numbers that will need costly medical and care services.
- Health promotion should be a top priority for policymakers.
- Information and education to promote healthy ageing across the course of people's lives from an early stage should be developed and disseminated as widely as possible.
- Policies and programmes need to be put in place to help halt the massive expansion of chronic disease.
- Need to focus on health promotion, disease prevention and increasing productivity.
- Need to support activities in early life that will enhance growth and development and prevent disease, e.g. obesity, osteoporosis, smoking.
- In adult life interventions are needed to prevent, reverse or slow down the onset of disease.
- In later life need to focus on maintaining independence, preventing and delaying disease and improving the quality of life for older people who live with some degree of illness or disability.
- Need to promote:
    - *Physical activity*
        - (i) regular, moderate exercise can delay functional decline and reduce the risk of chronic diseases in both healthy and chronically ill older people
        - (ii) it improves mental health and often promotes social contacts
        - (iii) being active can help older people maintain their activities of daily living as independently as possible for the longest period of time
        - (iv) there are economic benefits: medical costs are substantially lower.
    - *Healthy eating*
        - (i) malnutrition in older adults includes both under-nutrition and excess calorie consumption
        - (ii) obesity and a diet high in fat are related to conditions including cardiovascular disease and osteoarthritis
        - (iii) insufficient calcium and vitamin D intake is associated with a loss of bone density and consequently fractures.

- *Tobacco use*
  - (i) it is never too late to stop smoking
  - (ii) even in old age smoking cessation can reduce the rates of IHD, stroke and lung cancer.
- *Alcohol*
  - (i) older people are susceptible to alcohol-related diseases as well as being at risk of falls and injuries, and the potential hazards of mixing alcohol and medication.

- The determinants of active ageing:
  - *Social factors* – education/literacy/human rights/social support/prevention of violence and abuse
  - *Personal factors* – biology/genetics/adaptability
  - *Health/social services* – health promotion/disease prevention/long long-term care/primary care
  - *Physical environment* – urban and rural settings/housing/injury prevention
  - *Economic factors* – income/work/social protection
  - *Behavioural factors* – physical activity/healthy eating/cessation of tobacco use/control of alcohol problems/inappropriate use of medication.
- The health sector should:
  - reduce the burden of excess disability
  - reduce the risk factors associated with the causes of major diseases and increase the factors that protect health and wellbeing throughout the life course
  - develop primary healthcare systems that emphasise health promotion, disease prevention and the provision of cost-effective, equitable and dignified long-term care
  - advocate and collaborate with other sectors such as education, housing and employment to affect positive changes in the broad determinants of healthy active ageing.

2

Social processes in ageing

Introduction

Roles played by an individual over the life course may include:

- family roles (being son, daughter, wife, husband)
- social and community roles – neighbour, friend, etc.
- work roles.

These roles change throughout life and many decline after middle age. The impact of these changes varies from individual to individual and depends upon:

- the importance attached to them by the individual
- the importance attached to them by the society
- the individual's personality
- the individual's behaviour pattern
- the individual's financial circumstances in old age.

The three Rs that are said to define tasks of ageing and are associated with successful old age are:

1 accepting **reality** about one's capacities in health, social and financial realms
2 fulfilling **responsibilities** – planning for the survivors and making best choices regarding the remainder of life
3 exercising **rights** – right to live life as an individual at one's pace, right to privacy, right to respect, right to autonomy.

Despite the shift from extended family to nuclear family through mobility of families, size of housing and tendency for both partners to work, most older people still interact with their family and most have a relative living within travelling distance from them.

On the practical and positive side many older people fulfil an increasingly important role of grandparent through:

- providing of support in time of crisis
- babysitting
- providing income/financial support
- acting as confidant
- being a surrogate parent.

On the negative side many changes associated with ageing may be experienced as losses. These include:

- physical changes:
  - impaired vision
  - loss/reduction in hearing
  - decline in physical health.
- changes in social environment:
  - retirement (voluntary or involuntary)
  - reduced income
  - loss of social status
  - loss of social interaction
  - loss of personal standing/prestige
  - loss of home as a result of reduced income (about 40% of pensioners rely on means-tested benefit, and 50% receive at least three-quarters of their income from state benefits)
  - loss of privacy when forced to move into an institution.
- family changes:
  - with urbanisation extended family structure has been replaced by nuclear family
  - loss of family members and friends through death
  - strain on family relationship as a result of changes listed above and as a result of illness/disability.

Impact of social changes

Effects of these changes will depend on:

- individual's roles and habits in relation to members of family and society as a whole
- individual's health
- his/her behavioural capacities.

In some, these losses with the prospect of their own death may lead to bereavement and depression, while others may accept changes and achieve inner peace and self-acceptance, learn to tolerate the death of a spouse while developing new relationships, teaching others to live, passing on wisdom and finding a suitable living environment that allows maximum independence.

Family relationships

Family relationships, which provide an important focus for support to older people, are dependent upon/influenced by:

- previous closeness and supportiveness – satisfying in those who have had successful and close relationships. These individuals often feel they are successful in discharging an important obligation to a loved one. In others, resentment from the past may surface and lead to friction and psychological pain
- families being close and supportive – if they have not, it will not magically become so when parents become old and infirm. In fact resentment may surface
- extended family vs nuclear family
- whether older people themselves have to act as carers to their very old relatives
- changing role of females in society – a significant number are having to go out to work to support their own families and home
- health and dependency of an individual older person
- potential for large inheritance – in this situation rivalry may develop among family members. About 60% of older people over 65 are owner occupiers
- sibling position/relationship in a family – a rejected child may attempt to win love and recognition by helping the aged parents or may unconsciously punish them for rejection
- the parents' needs for assistance increase – children's attitudes may shift from affection to obligation
- actions/behaviours of an older person, e.g. playing manipulative games, using money to wield power, etc., which may/can lead to unhappy and angry children.

Relationship with onset of disability and illness

With onset of illness significant changes in family dynamics can take place, depending on previous family relationships. These include:

- increased stress/anxiety/tension
- disruption of usual interaction.

Caring, which in most cases is provided by a female relative, a spouse or a daughter, may lead to stress because of:

- time, effort and energy involved in care giving
- strain on job
- strain on own family
- loss of self-esteem
- depression and anger.

In managing illness in an older person family needs should be taken into consideration. Doctors should:

- ensure that the family feel they are actively involved
- provide information about the illness, provided the patient has given consent for this
- provide support and acknowledge their contribution.

Part II

Clinical aspects of old age

3

Age-associated physiological changes

Cross-sectional studies of ageing show that all physiological processes in general decline/deteriorate with age, although not all individuals will go through these changes at the same rate. Listed below are changes (anatomical and physiological) that have been described in cross-sectional studies and their likely impact.

Skin

Physical

- Fine wrinkling.
- Dryness.
- Laxity.
- Appearance of Campbell de Morgan spots.
- Cherry haemangiomas.
- Seborrhoeic keratosis.
- Greying of hairs due to reduction/loss of melanin from hair follicles.
- Brittle, slow-growing nails.

Histological

- Atrophy of epidermis.
- Fall in number of melanocytes.
- Reduction in Langerhans cells.
- Dermal fibroblasts.
- Loss of papillary dermal collagen.
- Thickened blood vessels.

- Reduction in mast cells.
- Reduction in number and function of sweat glands.
- Reduction in number of Pacinian and Meissner's corpuscles.

Gastrointestinal tract

The mouth

- Decrease in production of saliva.
- Impaired muscles of mastication.
- Tooth loss.
- Decrease in taste buds resulting in decrease in taste sensation.
- Decline in sense of smell.
- Enlargement of tongue.
- Atrophic changes in jaw.
- Senescent vascular lesions resembling those of hereditary haemorrhagic telangiectasia.

Possible impact of age-related changes. Changes in mastication as a result of dental changes; altered salivation and changes in efficiency of chewing due to muscular changes; impaired sense of smell and taste may lead to reduced food intake. This may be exacerbated by the decreased change in opioid and insulin receptors that influence appetite.

Upper GI tract

- Pharyngeal muscle weakness and abnormal relaxation of cricopharyngeal muscle.
- Reduced oesophageal peristalsis in the very elderly.
- Impaired relaxation of lower oesophageal sphincter.
- Increase in incidence of achlorhydria with age caused by chronic atrophic gastritis.

Small bowel

- Shortening and broadening of villi.

Possible impact. Impaired absorption/decreased efficiency in absorption, but this does not lead to clinical deficiencies.

Large bowel

- Atrophy of mucosa.
- Cell infiltration of lamina propria and mucosa.
- Hypertrophy of lamina muscularis mucosa.
- Increase in connective tissue.
- Atrophy of muscle layer.

Possible impact. Impaired motility/increased transit time with tendency to constipation, particularly in immobile older person.

Liver

- Decrease in liver volume – absolute and in relation to bodyweight.
- Decrease in liver blood flow.
- Fall in liver glycogen and ascorbic acid.

Impact. Decline in hepatic drug metabolism; however, conventional liver functions tests do not alter with age.

Gall bladder

- Hypertrophy of muscles but elasticity of wall may decrease.

Pancreas

- Deposition of amyloid in islets of Langerhans and blood vessels.
- Reduction in lipase but no change in amylase or bicarbonate.
- Duct hyperplasia.

Possible impact. Impaired fat absorption but not clinically significant.

Kidneys

- Reduction in size and weight of kidneys.
- Reduction in number and size of nephrons.
- Fall in number of glomeruli.
- Increase in sclerotic glomeruli.
- Loss of lobulation of glomerular tuft with thickening of membrane.

- Sclerotic changes in larger vessels.
- Degenerative changes in tubules.

Possible impact. Decline in glomerular filtration rate (decrease by 50% between the ages of 45 and 80) and impaired tubular function make an older person more susceptible to go into renal failure with dehydration or during an acute illness; dose of drugs which are primarily excreted by the kidneys may need adjustment in the elderly.

  NB: Renal function as measured by urea and creatinine reveals no abnormality in fit older person.

Bladder

- Increased incidence of trabeculation and pseudodiverticula.
- Changes in urethral epithelium to stratified squamous.
- Alteration in vascularity of submucosa.
- Decline in bladder capacity.
- In men there is tendency for prostate gland to enlarge with age.

Possible impact. These changes by themselves do not produce clinical symptoms but increase the likelihood of urinary tract infection developing.

Bone

- Bone loss (thinning of trabeculae and enlarged cancellous spaces) due to increased osteoclastic activity.
- Reduced ability to maintain matrix integrity.
- Fall in circulating hormones, such as growth hormone involved in maintaining tissue integrity.

Impact. Bone mass declines after middle age, with more marked decline during the first five years of menopause. By the age of 70, 50% of bone mass is lost in postmenopausal women, primarily due to fall in oestrogen level. Can be asymptomatic or lead to slight backache, kyphosis or stooped posture.

Cartilage of joints

- Breakdown of surface of cartilage (thinning, decrease in stiffness predisposing to osteoarthritis (OA)).

Heart

- Loss of myocytes in ventricles.
- Increase in interstitial fibrosis and collagen lead to increased stiffness of left ventricle.
- Deposition of amyloid, primarily in atria.
- Thickening of posterior left ventricular wall due to increase in volume.
- Increase in left atrial size.
- Increased stiffness of ventricles, thickening of the endocardium and valves.
- Increase in circulating catecholamines.
- Reduction in pacemaker cells in sinus node.

Blood vessels

- Thickening of smooth muscles in arterial wall – dilatation of large elastic arteries.
- Increase in systolic blood pressure due to increased stiffness of peripheral vessels and widened pulse pressure – this may impair left ventricular diastolic function.
- A slight decrease in diastolic blood pressure after the sixth decade.

Impact. 1 Prolonged myocardial contraction due to slow relaxation. 2 Reduction in resting stroke volume and cardiac output. 3 Decline in cardiovascular response to stress/exercise.

NB: While systolic function deteriorates on exercise, there is no reduction in resting LV ejection fraction; fourth heart sound may be heard in 60% of normal elderly; basal crackles may be present in immobile older person without heart failure; peripheral oedema may occur in immobile older person without heart failure.

Respiratory system

- Reduction in number of glandular epithelial cells – reduction in production of protective mucosa and impaired defence against infection.
- Changes in respiratory muscles – impaired strength and endurance.
- Ossification of costal cartilages, calcification of rib articulatory surfaces with muscular changes lead to impaired mobility of thoracic cage – fall in chest wall compliance.
- Thinning of alveoli.

- Lung volumes. Small increase in total lung capacity, large increase in functional residual capacity, fall in vital capacity, FEV_1, with a fall in FEV_1/FVC to a mean of 65% from age 70 and decline in maximal oxygen uptake.

Central nervous system changes

- Reduced brain weight – reduces after age 40–50 by 2–3% per decade.
- Brain shrinkage of overlying gyri.
- Thickening of meninges.
- Both grey and white matter decrease.
- Decline in nerve cell number, the greatest loss occurring in frontal and temporal cortices.
- Decrease in synaptic density in some areas.
- Plaques containing beta amyloid protein – found in over 70% of those over 80 years.
- Neurofibrillary tangles particularly in hippocampus and temporal cortex.
- Increase in CSF fluid spaces.

Impact. Age-related changes in pupils may be interpreted wrongly as indicating pathology; decreased density of pain receptors in skin – diminished sensitivity to light touch; altered pressure perception for one- or two-point discrimination; change in pain threshold; slowing of nerve conduction; decrease in ability to detect vibratory stimuli in fingers; tendon reflexes may be difficult to elicit and ankle jerk may be absent in normal older person as a result of age-related changes in sensory fibres.

Hearing

- Loss of hair cells in the cochlea.
- Loss of ganglion cells in the cochlea.
- Decrease in average number of fibres in the cochlear nerve.
- All these changes lead to presbyacusis, i.e. loss of hearing for high frequency sounds.

Eyes

- Flatter cornea leading to astigmatism.
- Hardening of lens and iris.

- Reduced response from ciliary muscles.
- Floaters in vitreous humour.
- Changes in skin and muscles leading to enophthalmos and ptosis – ptosis of upper eyelid seen in 11% of normal adults over age of 50.
- Small pupil – diameter of 1 mm or less commonly found in older persons.
- Pupils respond slowly to light.

Impact. Impaired near vision and astigmatism.

Lean body mass

- After the age of 40 lean body mass (LBM) falls, with rate of loss increasing with increasing age.
- Loss of number of muscle fibres plus possible reduction in size of remaining fibres and motor neurones.

Impact. Reduction in strength which may contribute to development of disability and falls. In addition one may note mild limb rigidity and paratonia.

Fat mass

Cross-sectional studies show increase in fat mass with age in both men and women; the increase in females is linear through to the eighth decade of life.

Aerobic capacity

Decreases in sedentary older people at the rate of 10% per decade. This of course can be increased by physical training in older people between the ages of 60 and 80.

Body temperature

- Impaired ability to maintain body temperature through thermogenesis.
- Impaired sweating, impaired shivering, impaired cutaneous vasoconstriction response to cold.
- Impaired perception of change in temperature.

Impact. These changes increase the older person's susceptibility to hypothermia.

Glucose homeostasis

In the elderly (60–90 years) insulin level rises sharply and then drops below the young adult mean – this is probably due to reduced sensitivity of muscles to insulin, insulin resistance and fall in insulin receptors in fat cells.

Impact. Impaired glucose tolerance test – plasma glucose rises to higher level and may remain elevated for longer. This is associated with a delay in rise of plasma insulin.

Hormonal changes

- *Reduced oestrogens.* Vaginal dryness, thinning of vaginal wall, vaginal shape – these changes may lead to pain and bleeding during coitus. In addition the changes in oestrogen lead to an increase in bone loss with the potential to produce osteoporosis.
- *Rise in FSH and LH.*
- *Adrenocortical function.* Basal, circadian rhythm and response to ACTH stimulation show no change with ageing.
- *Growth hormone.* Declines with age from a peak at about 30 years – decline being approximately 15% per decade. Decrease in circulating levels of insulin-like growth factor-I (IGF-I), a mediator through which GH produces its effects.
- *Thyroid.* With ageing it is common to find a decrease in size of follicles, progressive fibrosis and infiltration with lymphocytes. However, circulating free T4 and T3 do not change, except during an illness. In the very old elderly, i.e. over 80, thyroid activity may be low because of decrease in TSH and impairment of peripheral 5-deiodination. Impaired release of TSH – impaired TRH stimulation test.
- *PTH.* Serum levels rise with age. An older person has 30% higher levels than a young person. This correlates with decrease in vitamin D levels. These changes contribute to the age-related bone loss.

Blood

- Although there are bone marrow changes and the response of bone marrow to stimulation is reduced, there is little change in circulating cells with ageing.
- No change in levels of plasma coagulation factors.

Changes in immunity

- Increased immune deficiency, although variable, occurs and is due to decline in both cell-mediated and humoral immunity (reduction in active peripheral T cells with increase in immature T cells).
- Reduced T-cell response to interleukins and mitogens, reduction in the generation of cytotoxic T cells and humoral immunity (reduction in peak antibody response to immunisation and reduction in the duration of antibody response to immunisation).

Psychological changes

- Slowing of response to stimuli.
- Slowing of central processing information, i.e. slow response to cognitive tasks.
- Difficulties in developing concepts.
- Difficulty in thinking abstractly – better performance on concrete tasks.
- Become more rigid/less flexible.
- Curtail activities.
- Show increased reflectiveness.

Memory

- Require more time and effort to encode.
- Worsening of recall memory.

Intelligence

While cross-sectional studies suggest a decline with ageing, longitudinal data do not support this. More specifically, performance on verbal testing remains while performance on tests that require speed of response deteriorates with ageing.

Personality

Four personality types have been identified with ageing.

1   *Integrated individual.* 'Well-functioning', active person with intact cognitive abilities, is good organiser, flexible and satisfied with life. Some of these individuals voluntarily withdraw from role commitments and accept a

so-called 'rocking chair' approach to life – happy with the past and present and having little fear of the future.

2   *Armoured or defended individual.* Tries to fight the process of ageing and accepts each difficulty as a new challenge, but is often preoccupied with losses.

3   *The passive–dependent individual.* These individuals in their younger days were passive and apathetic and in old age have strong dependency needs and low level of life satisfaction. May have wish for death as they do not wish to be a burden.

4   *Angry individual.* This individual shows gross psychological pathology. The low activity and very low life satisfaction this individual experienced in younger days persist in old age and the person may often be bitter because of what they see as inequalities between old age and youth.

Stress and coping

The key factors that appear to have an impact on the individual's ability to cope with stresses associated with ageing as their role changes include financial resources, social and family supports, health, education, personality traits, religious belief and ability to develop specific coping strategies with stresses posed by retirement and bereavement.

4

Prevention of disease and disability

With increasing survival, many elderly patients can live 15–20 years beyond retirement and therefore prevention of disease is important. Furthermore, the increased level of disease and disability among the very old indicates that ways of preventing problems must be sought and implemented. The overall objective for the elderly should be to improve 'independent life expectancy'. Prevention may be classified as in Table 4.1.

Table 4.1: Classification of prevention

Primary
Prevention of disease occurrence (e.g. health promotion, immunisation)

Secondary
Early detection of disease (e.g. screening for cancers)

Tertiary
Prevention of complications of established disease (e.g. contractures after stroke)

Primary prevention

Health promotion

Health promotion comprises efforts to enhance positive health and prevent ill health through health education, illness prevention and environmental health. Advice on lifestyle modification such as stopping smoking, better diet and exercise is valuable for older as well as younger people. Other measures such as retirement training and bereavement counselling may also be important.

Social and economic factors

It is important to protect the living standards and disposable income of the elderly in order that they have access to healthy choices in lifestyle. Half of pensioner households depend on the state pension for 75% of their income and relative poverty shows a clear association with increased morbidity in terms of the number of chronic conditions and deteriorating functional status. It is important to identify and target disadvantaged groups such as ethnic minorities.

Diet

It is difficult for many elderly people to obtain an appropriate diet, due to limited income, limited access to transport and personal mobility problems. High prices in local shops, price differentials making 'healthy foods' more expensive and inappropriately packaged foods all contribute to making healthy choices more difficult for elderly people. Dietary counselling, especially at retirement, is effective in improving people's choice of healthy foods.

Exercise

Regular exercise improves strength, stamina, suppleness and wellbeing; however, the proportion of people taking regular exercise decreases with age. Regular appropriate exercise is associated with reduced cardiac and cerebrovascular disease, increased bone strength and a reduction in falls. Exercise needs to be continued for the benefits to be maintained. Health centres and local authorities increasingly offer active programmes to encourage the over-50s to take regular exercise. These need to be extended and tailored to meet the needs of the more frail elderly. In order to enjoy the benefits of exercise, some elderly patients may need chiropody, help with arthritis and pain relief, and reliable transport and these issues need to be addressed.

Accidents

There is an increasing risk of falls and accidents both in and outside the home with ageing. Poor lighting, environmental and domestic design, and personal factors such as decreasing visual acuity and balance are important factors. Recognised risk factors for recurrent falls include prescribed medication, lower limb disability, dementia and visual impairment. Along with increasing osteoporosis, especially in postmenopausal women, they lead to an increased rate of fractured neck of femur. Multifactorial intervention concentrating on medication adjustment, exercise programmes and adjusting the home environment can reduce the risk by 30%. Vitamin D and calcium supplementation can reduce fracture rates in nursing home patients and hip protectors reduce fracture rates in residential homes. Hormone replacement therapy (HRT) can reduce fracture rates following falls, but at present there are major concerns over the increased risk of breast cancer and cardiovascular and thrombotic disease associated with its use, so it is not currently recommended. The bisphosphonates also reduce fracture rates and are useful in those who can tolerate them.

Immunisation

Influenza and pneumonia cause high levels of morbidity and mortality in the elderly. Meta-analyses of 20 cohort studies involving 30 000 elderly patients show that influenza A and B vaccination reduces the risk of pneumonia and hospitalisation by 50% and death by 70%. Cost-benefit analysis in the UK has shown that immunisation should be offered to all people aged 65 and over and a target uptake of 70% has been set. Pneumococcal vaccination has a 50–80% efficacy in preventing pneumococcal bacteraemia in those over 65 years and those with chronic lung disease and heart disease. Vaccination should be offered to these groups and provides protection for 3–5 years.

Secondary prevention

Screening is the detection of disease at an early pre-symptomatic stage, before the patient would normally seek medical help. There is good evidence to support screening in the elderly, but unfortunately policy does not always accord with scientific evidence and the elderly are often not included in screening programmes. In practice, the benefits are likely to be at least as great, if not greater, among elderly than among young people. It is important to recognise the difference between screening and case finding. Screening aims to measure all eligible people, whereas case finding is the opportunistic detection of disease or problems, usually when patients attend the surgery, often with another problem. The cost and ethical aspects of the two approaches are very different. Case finding is relatively cheap and raises few ethical issues. Screening is more expensive and implies that the services are sufficient to deal with all the problems detected. Some examples where screening is beneficial follow.

- Treatment of hypertension has been shown to reduce the risk of stroke by up to 75%. As the risk of stroke increases dramatically with age, many more strokes will be prevented by treatment of hypertension in the elderly, compared to young adults who have a low risk of stroke.
- Statins are effective lipid-lowering drugs and recent trials have shown that the beneficial effects in primary and secondary prevention are evident in older patients.
- Aspirin and warfarin are beneficial in reducing stroke in patients with atrial fibrillation, but are often not prescribed for elderly patients in spite of the fact that both conditions are more common in the elderly.
- Despite evidence to support mammography and cervical smear screening in older women, these services are not offered to women over the age of 65, although they can request a test.
- The benefits of screening for prostate and colorectal cancers in the UK remain unclear, but have been endorsed in the US.
- Simple measures for checking visual acuity, screening for glaucoma, hearing, dental and locomotor activity would make a significant contribution to the quality of life of older people if coupled to ease of access to corrective procedures of known effectiveness.

Tertiary prevention

In many cases this is detecting disease that, although symptomatic, is largely unrecognised or under-reported. Elderly patients are more likely to have covert problems that are attributed to the ageing process by both patients and health professionals. The 1990 GP Contract required GPs to offer an annual visit to every person over 75 years to assess the following problems:

- visual and hearing impairments
- immobility
- mental conditions (depression and dementia)
- physical conditions (incontinence)
- use of medications.

All of these problems are common in the elderly, but there is a significant shortfall in the diagnosis of these disorders. Early detection and treatment of these problems should improve the patient's physical, mental and social wellbeing.

A number of treatments for established disease have been shown to be beneficial in the elderly. Such areas include hip replacement surgery, treatment of coronary heart disease (CHD), valve replacement, general surgery and anti-cholinesterases in dementia. Unfortunately many elderly people still do not have equity of access to these important therapies, which have been shown to improve their quality of life.

5

Specific features of disease presentation

While an older person as well as a younger person can exhibit clinical features that lead to a unifying single diagnosis, a significant number do not. The differences between these sick old people and younger persons can be summarised by the helpful mnemonic 'NAMES'.

- **N**on-specific presentation.
- **A**typical or uncommon presentation.
- **M**ultiple pathologies or diagnoses.
- **E**rroneous attribution of symptoms to old age.
- **S**ingle pathology/illness can lead to catastrophic consequences.

Non-specific presentation

The non-specific presentation has been described in terms of 'dragons' by the first President of the British Geriatrics Society, Dr Trevor Howell and as 'giants of geriatric medicine' by Professor Bernard Isaacs. Recently geriatricians have tried to fit the pattern of presentation into an aide-memoire using the letter 'I'.

'Dragons'	'Giants of geriatric medicine'	'Is'
Confusion	Confusion	Intellectual failure
Incontinence	Incontinence	Incontinence
Contractures of joint	Immobility	Immobility
Bedsores and other ulcers	Falls	Instability
Falls		Iatrogenic illness

With such non-specific presentation differential diagnosis in a sick older person can be broad and the doctor has to use all available information from the history (which may have to be sought from a third party) and carry out a full examination and appropriate investigations to find the cause of vague symptoms.

Atypical or uncommon presentation

Atypical or uncommon symptoms may replace the commonly stated/quoted features of illness, for example:

- myocardial infarction, instead of producing central crushing chest pain with radiation into the left arm or the neck, may present with shortness of breath or a fall resulting from a cardiac arrhythmia or hypotension or with confusion
- pneumonia or other serious infections may not give rise to an elevated white cell count or rise in temperature
- peptic ulcer perforation in an older person can be asymptomatic and may not produce the classic rigid abdomen with rebound tenderness, and the diagnosis may be made by examination of the chest x-ray
- psychiatric illness may present with vague physical symptoms or multiple somatic complaints
- apathetic thyrotoxicosis, silent pulmonary embolism
- heart failure without dyspnoea.

Multiple pathologies

With ageing there is an increasing tendency for many pathologies, which increases the risk of iatrogenic illness in old age. The main factors that contribute to the development of multiple diseases in the elderly include:

1 increase in age-related incidence of common disorders, e.g. hypertension, osteoarthritis, diabetes mellitus, vascular disease, dementia
2 impaired immune system leading to increased chances of cancer and hypothyroidism
3 increased likelihood of an illness affecting one system leading to disorder in another, e.g. respiratory infection leading to development of atrial fibrillation and heart failure
4 vascular diseases may develop gradually and during the latent period acute illness may develop in an older individual

5 immobility associated with many neurological or musculoskeletal disorders may lead to an increased risk of developing complications such as falls, urinary incontinence, infections, pressure sores, deep vein thrombosis plus pulmonary embolism.

Erroneous attribution of symptoms in old age

Doctors as well as elderly people themselves may mistakenly attribute non-specific signs and symptoms to old age. It is not uncommon to hear an elderly person say 'It is my age, doctor' or 'I am only here because my son or daughter is worried'. One of the reasons for an elderly person not presenting early with symptoms is denial, fear of what might be found.

Single illness/pathology leading to catastrophic consequences

While in a young person a simple illness (such as an influenza) may produce symptoms that last for a few days, in some older people it can lead to a cascade of events with dire consequences (*see* Figure 5.1).

Other consequences of illness in old age

- Apart from abnormality of one or more organs of the body, an illness has other consequences for the individual as a whole, leading to physical, psychological, functional and social problems.
- The impairments, disabilities and handicaps associated with the illness in an older person require full and thorough assessments, not only from a physician but from other professionals, whose roles are to develop and implement rehabilitation in order to achieve maximum recovery and function.
- If handicap or disability cannot be abolished, then the team tries to ensure that an individual is able to live as independent a life as possible with support of individuals or aids and adaptations and services that meet their needs (*see* Chapter 7).
- In attempting to meet the physical and psychological needs of an individual, professionals try to reduce the individual's distress, improve their

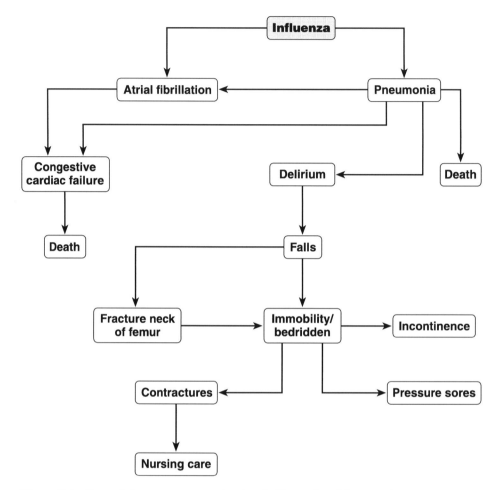

Figure 5.1   Potential consequences of a simple illness for older people.
Reproduced from *Elderly Medicine: A training guide* edited by Gurcharan S Rai and
Graham P Mulley. By permission of Martin Dunitz, Andover.

wellbeing and quality of life (people themselves are the best judges of
what makes 'life worth living').

Physical signs and old age

Age-related changes may lead to physical signs or may influence the sensitivity of physical signs in indicating the presence of a disease process.
Examples of these include:

1 small pupils that respond sluggishly to light
2 changes in eyelids producing ptosis

3   absent ankle jerks
4   reduced vibration sensation in fingers
5   displaced apex beat due to the presence of kyphoscoliosis
6   presence of pulmonary crackles in the absence of cardiac or pulmonary disease in the immobile older person.

Further reading

- Hodkinson HM (1973) Non-specific presentation of illness. *BMJ*. **4**: 94.
- Horan MA (1998) Introduction – presentation of disease in old age. In: JC Brocklehurst, RC Tallis and HM Fillit (eds) *Textbook of Geriatric Medicine & Gerontology*. Churchill Livingstone, Edinburgh.
- Isaacs B, Livingstone M and Neville Y (1972) *Survival of the Unfittest*. Routledge & Kegan Paul, London.

6

Pharmacology and therapeutics

Older people receive more prescriptions per head than any other group and 45% of NHS prescribing is for people over 65 years of age. Prescribing for the elderly is complex. Because chronic illness increases with advancing age, older people are more likely to have conditions that require drug treatment. The recognition that primary and secondary prevention therapies benefit older as much as younger patients has added to the need for multiple medication. However, the hazards of prescribing many drugs, including side-effects, drug interactions and difficulties of compliance, are also particular problems in the elderly.

The RCP report *Medication for Older People*[1] indicated that excessive prescribing was widespread in the elderly and recommended careful consideration as to whether drug treatment was appropriate. The National Service Framework (NSF) for Older People[2] has prioritised the need for appropriate and rational prescribing for elderly patients, acknowledging the problems of polypharmacy, but highlighting that medicines are also underused in the elderly and identifying the need for linking prescribing data with clinical data.

Proper use of medication in the elderly has beneficial effects and improves functional status. Therefore, elderly patients should not be denied medication on the basis of age. There is evidence that older patients are underprescribed useful drugs, including aspirin for secondary prevention in high-risk patients, beta-blockers following myocardial infarction and warfarin for non-valvular atrial fibrillation. It is acknowledged that there is often a delay between publication and application of the results in clinical practice. However, even when published data are known for a number of years and receive considerable attention in the medical press, there is evidence of underprescribing in the elderly. There is also evidence that the elderly receive medications that could potentially cause more harm than good. A key difference in distinguishing appropriate from inappropriate drug use is evident in the themes of polymedicine and polypharmacy. Polymedicine describes the use of medications for the treatment of multiple co-morbid conditions, while polypharmacy represents a less than desirable state with duplicated medications, drug-to-drug interactions, and inadequate attention paid to pharmacokinetic and pharmacodynamic principles. Finding the right balance between too few and too many drugs will help ensure increased longevity, improved overall health, and enhanced functioning and quality of life for the ageing population.

Adverse drug reactions

Drug-related illness is a significant problem in the elderly. From 5% to 17% of hospital admissions are caused by adverse reactions to medicines and 6–17% of older patients in hospital experience adverse drug reactions.[2] The risk of an adverse effect with a drug increases with age and the number of drugs prescribed. Several mechanisms may account for this, including:

- altered pharmacokinetics and pharmacodynamics with age (see below)
- increased sensitivity of diseased tissue to drug toxicity
- potential drug interactions
- difficulties in patient compliance with an increasing number of drugs
- prescription of drugs that are unnecessary for the treatment of ailments that might be better managed through non-pharmacological means
- inappropriate prescription of drugs that are either contraindicated or prescribed in combination with other drugs that produce potential drug interactions.

Drug–drug interactions constitute only a small proportion of adverse drug reactions and are important because they are often predictable and therefore avoidable. The most important mechanisms for drug–drug interactions are the inhibition or induction of drug metabolism, and pharmacodynamic potentiation or antagonism. Interactions involving a loss of action of one of the drugs are at least as frequent as those involving an increased effect. It is likely that only about 10% of potential interactions result in clinically significant events and, while death or serious clinical consequences are rare, low-grade, clinically unspectacular morbidity in the elderly may be much more common. Non-specific complaints (e.g. confusion, lethargy, weakness, dizziness, incontinence, depression, falling) should all prompt a closer look at the patient's drug list.

Alterations to pharmacokinetics and pharmacodynamics with ageing

Knowledge of the interplay between ageing physiology, chronic diseases and drugs will help avoid potential adverse drug events as well as drug–drug and drug–disease interactions. Despite the relative paucity of drug trials in the old and especially the very old (over 85 years), some general principles of pharmacology in the ageing patient can be taken from available data and clinical experience. The pharmacokinetic changes most consistently seen with ageing occur in the volume of distribution, clearance and half-life of a drug.

- Renal drug clearance is consistently diminished with ageing.
- Hepatic metabolism is more variably affected and, in contrast to renal clearance, no reliable formula exists to estimate hepatic drug clearance.
- The absorption of drugs is generally unchanged with the exception of drugs that are metabolised to active compounds by the liver. In this case absorption is increased, leading to greater bioavailability and greater effect.
- The volume of distribution of a drug depends on whether it is water soluble or lipid soluble. With age the ratio of fat to lean muscle increases; therefore lipid soluble drugs such as benzodiazepines have an increased volume of distribution leading to prolonged effects, and water-soluble drugs such as alcohol and digoxin have a smaller volume of distribution, leading to more rapid peak effects.
- Alteration in receptor response may lead to increased or decreased drug effects.

These changes in pharmacokinetics and pharmacodynamics may result in a prolonged drug half-life, an increased potential for drug toxicity and a greater likelihood for adverse drug reactions.

Better prescribing in the elderly

Drug-related morbidity and mortality is an important area to target, both to improve the quality of medical care for elderly people and to reduce the costs of healthcare for this population. There are a number of strategies that can be adopted to decrease the risk of potential clinical problems.

- The number of drugs prescribed for each individual should be limited to as few as is necessary.
- The use of drugs should be reviewed regularly and unnecessary agents withdrawn if possible, with subsequent monitoring.
- Drugs should be started in reduced doses with slow incremental increases and close monitoring for drug interactions and adverse drug reactions.
- Patients should be encouraged to alert physicians, pharmacists and other healthcare professionals to symptoms that occur when new drugs are introduced.

- Physicians with a responsibility for elderly people in an institutional setting should develop a strategy for monitoring their drug treatment.
- For those adverse drug reactions that come to clinical attention, it is important to review why they happened and to plan for future prevention.
- Clinicians should report, via the appropriate postmarketing surveillance scheme, any adverse drug reactions they have encountered.
- Multidisciplinary education about the nature of physiological ageing and its effect on drug handling, and the possible presentations of drug-related disease in older patients is required.

Compliance

Poor compliance with medication is also an important problem in the elderly, occurring in 40–75% of prescriptions, and the consequences may be serious. Some common forms of drug treatment non-compliance are found in the elderly: overuse and abuse, forgetting, and alteration of schedules and doses.

- Some older patients who are acutely ill may take more than the prescribed dose of a medication in the mistaken belief that more of the drug will speed their recovery. Such overuse has clearly been associated with adverse drug effects.
- Forgetting to take a medication is a common problem in older people and is especially likely when an older patient takes several drugs simultaneously. Data suggest that the use of three or more drugs a day places elderly people at particular risk of poor compliance. As many as 25% of older people take at least three drugs and elderly hospitalised patients typically take eight drugs simultaneously. Problems may also arise when dementia or depression is present, which may interfere with memory.
- The most common non-compliant behaviour of the elderly appears to be underuse of the prescribed drug. Inappropriate drug discontinuation may occur in up to 40% of prescriptions, mostly within the first year.
- As many as 10% of elderly people may take drugs prescribed for others and more than 20% may take drugs not currently prescribed by a physician.

Compliance with medication can be improved by careful explanation of the reasons for treatment, expected drug effects and side-effects, use of tablet cards, pill holders and better labelling of medication. Recent studies in heart failure have shown that nurse specialists can improve compliance in the elderly and reduce mortality and morbidity.

Key points

▼ Whenever possible, alternatives to medication therapy should be considered as the initial treatment of choice in the elderly.

▼ Medications should be prescribed when indicated and not withheld due to a patient's age.

▼ Start with low doses and simplify dose and drug regimens.

▼ Keep the number of medications to the minimum possible to reduce the risk of adverse drug reactions and drug-to-drug interactions.

▼ Review medication regularly and especially prior to initiating new therapy.

▼ Explain why the medication is needed and what effects and side-effects are to be expected.

▼ Follow-up care to review the efficacy and monitor any potential side-effects is crucial.

▼ Timely discontinuation of a drug when therapeutic usefulness is past is equally important.

References

1 Royal College of Physicians (1997) *Medication for Older People* (2e). Royal College of Physicians, London.
2 Department of Health (2001) *National Service Framework for Older People. Medicines and Older People*. Department of Health, London.

7

Principles of rehabilitation

The World Health Organization (WHO) has defined rehabilitation as an active process by which those people who are disabled by injury or disease achieve a full recovery or realise their optimal physical, mental and social potential and are integrated into their most appropriate environment.

Definition of impairment, disability and handicap

- *Impairment* is a loss or abnormality of psychological, physiological or anatomical structure or function.
- *Disability* is any restriction or lack of ability to perform a task or activity within the range considered as normal activity.
- *Handicap* is the social disadvantage suffered by an individual as a result of ill health compared to a normal person of the same age, sex and background.

Rehabilitation is a complex process and requires a skilled team with effective leadership. Success is usually measured in terms of the extent to which a person returns to a normal lifestyle. In many cases successful rehabilitation may mean some degree of acceptance of disability by the patient, and provision of some alternative means of achieving tasks that cannot be done independently. Rehabilitation is an important factor in elderly care medicine as:

- acute illness in older people often has functional consequences (especially mobility and self-care)
- many degenerative disease processes (osteoarthritis, ischaemic heart disease, peripheral vascular disease, chronic lung disease, stroke, osteoporosis and fractured neck of femur) are age related
- the prevalence of disability increases with age.

The principles of rehabilitation and the processes involved in the elderly are outlined in Tables 7.1 and 7.2.

Table 7.1:   Key principles of rehabilitation in the elderly

Wholeness	Address the whole person rather than a part
Individualised	
Emphasis on functional abilities	Self-care, mobility, life spaces and leisure
Not time limited	Wider vision than hospital care
Active, planned responses	Requires a creative problem-solving approach

Table 7.2:   The clinical process of rehabilitation

Key tasks	Processes used
Recognition of potential	Multidisciplinary team assessment
Rehabilitation goal setting	Multidisciplinary team meeting
Re-ablement	General and special techniques
Regular review	Further assessment
Resettlement	Home visits, follow-up, liaison with primary care team
Readjustment	Empowering by education about disability and available services

Rehabilitation goals are highly focused statements of intent that should be generated from the assessment process and then agreed. Using goals has been shown to lead to improved outcomes provided that significant patient involvement occurs, and that both short- and long-term goals are developed. Goals need to be **S**pecific, **M**easurable, **A**chievable, **R**ealistic and **T**imed (SMART).

There are a number of systematic reviews for rehabilitation topics of relevance to the elderly, including falls, fractured neck of femur, stroke, etc. Most studies describe the effects of complex, multi-component interventions, but in many cases the critical factor for successful rehabilitation remains undefined.

Stroke rehabilitation

Recovery from stroke occurs over at least three months, and in some cases may continue for over one year. Little research has been done on later recovery, but measurable recovery beyond a year is probably uncommon. The spontaneous recovery is due to resolution of cerebral oedema surrounding the damaged brain, and relearning of skills. Rehabilitation should start from day one, though initially this may be mainly concerned with putting joints through a passive range of movements, giving advice on lifting and handling the patient, and helping with positioning of limbs and trunk.

There is now considerable evidence from clinical trials showing that patients managed in an organised stroke unit are more likely to survive, return home and regain independence than those who receive conventional care on a general ward. Various models of stroke care have been tested, but they all have the following features in common:

- co-ordinated interdisciplinary team care
- ability to provide rehabilitation for several weeks if necessary
- staff with interest in stroke/rehabilitation
- education programmes and training in stroke.

Much of the management of the stroke patient incorporates an inter-disciplinary process in which a number of disciplines may carry out a number of assessments and identify a range of problems. The interdisciplinary process involves a goal-planning cycle in which the patient is assessed, a problem is identified, a recovery goal is set, an intervention is provided and then the process is reassessed. This process can occur on several timescales and involve both short- and long-term goals. Close co-operation and liaison are essential to ensure compatible goals and objectives. The first step is to achieve reasonable sitting balance, then move on to standing and transfers, and then to walking. Reassessment is essential to identify progress and define any potential barriers to successful rehabilitation, which may be physical (e.g. pneumonia), psychological (e.g. depression), social (e.g. unsuitable housing) or cultural (e.g. patients' and/or families' reaction to disability).

The key members of the interdisciplinary team include the following.

- *Doctors* need to have knowledge of the diagnosis, prognosis and complications of stroke.
- *Nurses* play a central role, providing for the daily needs of patients, preventing complications, providing regular assessments of progress and support for patients and family.
- *Physiotherapists* are largely concerned with the recovery of movement and are involved in assessing motor and sensory function, advising and managing position and handling issues, training in walking and the provision of aids, and preventing complications (especially respiratory).
- *Occupational therapists* play a key role in the recovery of functional tasks. They provide detailed assessments of activities of daily living and other aspects of occupational performance, including assessing visuo-spatial function, providing aids and appliances, and assessing patients' abilities within the home setting.

- *Speech and language therapists* – swallowing difficulties affect up to one-third of patients after stroke and it is vital that this is recognised and that speech therapists are involved early in the management of these patients. Often recovery takes a week or two and all that is required is careful feeding and thickened fluids. In more severe cases it is necessary to use a nasogastric tube for feeding and if the problem persists, a feeding gastrostomy may be required for long-term management. Impairment of speech is devastating to most patients. Speech therapists can help make the best use of whatever modalities of communication remain and advise family and staff about how best to communicate. Correction of other impairments such as deafness or reduced sight can often aid communication.
- *Clinical psychologists* are frequently involved in managing psychological and behavioural complications of stroke.
- *Social workers* help access services and facilities within a community setting.
- *Dieticians* advise on the management of nutritional problems and feeding regimens for enteral feeding.
- *Psychiatrists* advise on the management of affective complications of stroke.
- *Ophthalmologists* help in the management of patients with visual problems.

The outcome of rehabilitation is dependent on a number of factors including:

- severity of initial deficit (Table 7.3)
- extreme frailty
- premorbid functional level
- haemorrhagic rather than ischaemic stroke
- prolonged drowsiness
- depression
- presence of intercurrent disease and other co-morbidities such as cardiac failure
- location of the stroke: infarction of the non-dominant hemisphere may produce unilateral neglect, visuo-spatial and topographical disorientation, which will influence recovery and function; dysphasic patients with severely limited comprehension also have particular problems. Extensive cortical sensory loss is also regarded as a poor prognostic sign and more subtle defects that adversely affect outlook include intellectual impairment, apraxia, denial, impaired memory and motor perseveration.

Table 7.3:   Markers of stroke severity

Unconscious during the first 24 hours
Incontinence of urine
Perceptual impairments
Loss of proprioception
Cognitive impairment

Lower limb amputee rehabilitation

The average age of people undergoing lower limb amputation is 70 and 25% are over 80 years of age. The majority have peripheral vascular and may have associated cardiovascular disease, cerebrovascular disease, chronic lung disease and diabetes. The loss of a limb in the elderly seriously threatens independence. Successful rehabilitation is most likely when a single person, either a rehabilitation consultant, a vascular surgeon or a geriatrician, co-ordinates and is responsible for the programme.

Rehabilitation after lower limb amputation typically involves three stages.

1 *Preoperative assessment.* The patient should be referred to a physiotherapist ideally several weeks preoperatively. This allows time to improve strength in the other limbs and to optimise mobility and functional status. The physio-therapist can also inform the patient and carers of the probable rehabilitation programme and expected outcome.
2 *Postoperative care.* Initial physical therapy is aimed at stabilising residual limb volume by decreasing oedema and promoting healing. The use of early walking aids improves functional recovery. A typical programme would include:
   - Days 1–3: bed exercises to strengthen arms, abdominal muscles, lower back and remaining leg and balance training in the sitting position. A full range of hip and knee extension is required to maintain joint mobility and avoid contractures
   - Days 4–6: training in transfers from bed to chair and wheelchair mobility is initiated. Balance and walking training with a walking frame is started
   - Days 7–10: an early walking aid such as a pneumatic post-amputation aid is introduced, initially twice daily for 10 minutes increasing to one hour twice daily over 1–2 weeks.
3 *Prosthetic programme.* A prosthesis should be fitted if possible, even in the presence of other limiting medical conditions, as it facilitates transfers and standing and has added cosmetic value. Some older patients decline the

offer of a prosthetic programme and opt for wheelchair mobility. Limb fitting usually begins about three weeks postoperatively after below-knee amputation, provided wound healing is satisfactory. Prosthetic training focuses on stump care and bandaging, transferring and hopping with use of an aid. The programme then continues where feasible with improving balance and general fitness and walking on slopes and rough ground. Unfortunately the energy expenditure required for mobilising with an above-knee amputation is beyond the capacity of many elderly patients, especially those with cardiorespiratory problems. Nonetheless, with appropriate rehabilitation and social support the majority of elderly amputees return home and lead functionally useful lives.

The functional outcome of rehabilitation in lower limb amputation depends on a number of factors including:

- the level of amputation
- premorbid health (especially cardiovascular status)
- co-morbidities
- psychosocial factors
- patient motivation.

Other factors that can affect rehabilitation progress include stump pain, phantom sensations and phantom pain. In addition, elderly amputees are a high-risk group with up to 50% dying within the next three years, often as a result of cardiovascular or cerebrovascular disease. Furthermore, 25% of non-diabetics and 50% of diabetics require another amputation within the next five years.

Rehabilitation in rheumatic and orthopaedic disorders

Arthritis and other rheumatic disorders are among the most prevalent chronic health problems in the elderly and often lead to compromised function, falls and loss of independence. Difficulties with mobility, upper extremity function, household management and self-care activities are associated with joint pain and arthritis. Effective management of arthritis in older people should include concurrent pharmacological and non-pharmacological interventions with targeted goals of pain relief, preservation of functional independence and quality of life. The American College of Rheumatology (ACR) guidelines (1995) for the management of hip and knee arthritis highlight the importance of non-pharmacological measures to relieve pain, and improve joint biomechanics and overall function (Table 7.4).

Table 7.4:   Management of osteoarthritis (ACR guidelines, 1995)[1]

Non-pharmacological	Pharmacological
To relieve pain Ice, heat, ultrasound, TENS	• Analgesic medication • Topical salicylate or capsaicin • Adjunctive agents (tricyclic antidepressants)
To relieve pain and improve joint mechanics • Mobility aids (sticks, frame, etc.) • Orthotic devices • Weight reduction if obese	Arthrocentesis with intra-articular glucocorticoids
To improve muscle strength and conditioning • Physical therapy • Resistive exercise training • Aerobic conditioning	
Pain still limiting function in spite of maximal therapy Chronic pain management if unsuitable for surgery	Surgical evaluation

Physiotherapists play an important role in management of the patient with arthritis and rheumatism and can:

- assess joint function and associated limitations
- advise on and supervise exercise programmes to improve joint biomechanics and mobility. Resistive training and aerobic exercises have been shown to improve physical performance, painful symptoms and reports of disability after three months
- use physical therapy such as ice, heat, ultrasound and TENS to relieve pain
- advise on aerobic exercise to assist weight loss.

Occupational therapists can:

- assess functional limitations
- provide therapy to maintain and/or improve function
- advise on aids and adaptations to facilitate independence.

Podiatrists may also be involved and can:

- advise on orthotic devices and shock-absorbing shoes that have been shown to compensate for functional defects and are protective.

Dieticians provide:

- dietary advice to the obese patient as weight reduction may significantly reduce pain by reducing biomechanical stress on weight-bearing joints.

Rehabilitation after hip fracture

Hip fracture is common in the elderly with annual rates per 1000 of 2–3 for men and 3–6 for women aged 65–74 years, and 15–20 for men and 25–40 for women over 85 years of age. The one-year mortality rate after hip fracture is about 30% and a significant proportion fail to regain their previous functional level. Co-morbidities are common. Rehabilitation needs to commence as soon as possible after surgery to promote independent mobility and function, and collaboration between orthopaedic surgeons, geriatricians and other members of the multidisciplinary team is essential to assist medical management and rehabilitation. Early rehabilitation after hip fracture focuses on prevention of deep venous thrombosis, pressure sores, pneumonia and atelectasis, and constipation.

- *Physiotherapy* should start on day one post-surgery with careful assessment of hip movement. An active range of movement of the unaffected leg together with isometric exercises of the quadriceps and gluteals of the affected leg are begun. On day two, transfers and bed mobility are taught and assisted standing can occur in most patients. From day three the patient can start to walk short distances with a standard walking frame. Decisions on weight bearing depend on the type of fixation, bone quality, fracture location and the patient's cognitive and functional ability to comply with graded degrees of weight bearing. In most patients weight bearing with a standard walking frame is possible in the first week after surgery, but this may be delayed if fixation is less secure or there is severe osteoporosis. During week two the patient can usually progress to a wheeled walker that allows faster walking and an improved gait pattern. Later the patient can progress to a stick held in the opposite hand. To avoid posterior dislocation a number of precautions are necessary, including avoiding hip flexion of over 90°, leg adduction past the mid-line and combined movements such as flexion and internal rotation. Exercise programmes to improve balance and co-ordination should be undertaken in the longer term to reduce the risk of further falls.
- *Occupation therapists* also play an important role in assessing and improving functional activities to facilitate independent living.
- *Dieticians* are essential as many elderly patients with fractured hips are malnourished and this can adversely affect the outcome of rehabilitation.

Factors influencing the outcome of rehabilitation after fractured neck of femur include:

- preoperative functional ability
- co-morbidities
- cognitive impairment.

Reference

1 Hochberg MC, Altman RG, Branett D *et al.* (1995) Guidelines for the medical management of osteoarthritis of the hip and the knee. *Arthritis & Rheumatism.* **38**(11): 1535–46.

Further reading

- Mulley G (1994) The principles of rehabilitation. *Rev Clin Gerontol.* **4**: 61–9.
- Royal College of Physicians (2004) *National Clinical Guidelines for Stroke* (2e). Royal College of Physicians, London. www.rcplondon.ac.uk
- SIGN (2002) *Management of Patients with Stroke. Rehabilitation, prevention and management of complications and discharge planning.* SIGN Guideline No. 64. www. sign.ac.uk

8

Domiciliary care for disabled older people

Given the high prevalence of chronic disease in the elderly, disability is a common problem. The majority of frail and disabled elderly people, including those with severe functional impairment, live in private households. Organising services for these patients requires careful assessment by a team approach to determine disease processes, functional ability, continence, cognition, mobility and social background. The National Health Service and Community Care Act (1990) gave local authority social service departments the lead responsibility for assessing individual need and planning, delivering and monitoring care for elderly and disabled people. The main objectives of the Act are:

- to promote domiciliary, day and respite services to enable older people to live in their own homes wherever possible
- to provide practical support to carers, such as financial help and information about services
- to assess need and have good management to ensure high-quality care
- to promote the development of independent care providers
- to clarify the responsibilities of care agencies; community care plans should show who is responsible for which services
- to secure better value for taxpayers' money.

The characteristics and range of services provided by the different agencies are summarised in Table 8.1. In the past local authorities were the major providers of services for the elderly, but increasingly the independent sector plays a greater part in providing basic services like meals, home helps and respite care.

Table 8.1:   Summary of services provided for elderly patients in the community

	Services provided
Informal carers	Personal hygiene Domestic tasks Nursing tasks Financial help Counselling
Local authority social services	Home help Meals on wheels Social worker Respite care Occupational therapy Day centres Lunch clubs
Local health services	General practitioner District nurses Palliative care MacMillan nursing Pharmacist Podiatry Therapists (physiotherapy/speech and language) Dietician Continence advisory services Dental care Opticians Audiology services
Private services	Home care services Meals on wheels Respite care Nursing and residential homes Domiciliary nursing services Live-in companions
Voluntary services	National organisations (e.g. Age Concern, Help the Aged) Disease- or disability-specific organisations (e.g. Arthritis Council, Parkinson's Disease Society, Alzheimer's Disease Society) Organisations for carers (Crossroads, Carers National Association) Locally oriented organisations (Citizens Advice Bureau, Women's Royal Voluntary Service) Culturally based services Lunch clubs Day centres Hospices Housing associations

Informal carers, including family, friends and neighbours, provide a significant amount of the care. They are readily available and flexible and able to deal with unexpected events and emergencies. However, there is little recognised training or support for informal carers, many of whom are elderly and have their own health problems and they are often expected to do a job that few health professionals would consider feasible. It is important to recognise that informal carers need training to carry out many of the tasks of assisting disabled people. The best training is one-to-one with a therapist and carried out in the patient's home if possible.

Formal agencies have a larger pool of people and a range of technical expertise, skill and resources that may be essential for the patient, but are often less flexible and less available than informal carers.

Equipment

A number of different aids and appliances are available that may help maintain functional ability, including:

- hoists and transfer boards assist with lifting
- walking sticks, crutches, frames and wheelchairs assist in maintaining mobility
- battery-operated wheelchairs and tricycles are expensive, but help maintain outdoor mobility
- stairlifts are expensive, but may be valuable for some patients.

Given the individual nature of disability it is often difficult to determine what will suit a particular patient. A major difficulty in deciding what would be useful is the limited opportunity to test pieces of equipment, especially if they are expensive. Joint assessment by a physiotherapist and occupational therapist is the best way of ensuring the patient gets the right aids for both lifting and transfers and mobility.

Services

- *Respite care* is used mainly to give carers a break from the burden of caring. It is a limited resource and, even when available, may be underused by carers who often find it difficult to accept their own needs for support and respite. Respite is usually provided in residential or nursing homes, depending on the physical and mental condition of the patient. Respite should be used as a valuable opportunity to reassess the patient and, where appropriate, provide treatment aimed at maintaining function.

- *Podiatry services.* Elderly patients often require the services of a podiatrist. Even simple problems like uncut nails and corns can render a patient housebound and immobile. The podiatrist can also treat congenital and acquired foot problems and recognise pedal manifestations of systemic disease such as vascular disease and peripheral neuropathy. Unfortunately, there are insufficient numbers of podiatrists to provide an adequate service to the elderly, many of whom are housebound and require domiciliary care.
- *Community psychiatric nurses* assess, treat and monitor all aspects of psychiatric illness, including dementia in the elderly, and liaise closely with consultant psychogeriatricians. They also have roles in education both with the patient and carer and support both, thereby playing an important role in maintaining mentally ill elderly people in the community.
- *Continence advisors* are experts in the management of both urinary and faecal incontinence and give specific advice on the continence aids available as well as their use by the patient and/or carer.
- *Dieticians.* Malnutrition is not infrequent in the elderly and is often unrecognised. Dieticians can assess and treat patients and provide valuable advice, especially in patients with swallowing difficulties who may have problems meeting their nutritional needs either orally or by enteral feeding.
- *Audiology services.* Hearing loss is common, affecting one in three of the elderly, and can lead to withdrawal from society. Patients should be referred to an audiology clinic for assessment. The standard approach is to issue a hearing aid, but elderly patients often find these of little help or are unable to use them properly due to problems with manual dexterity, etc. Malfunctioning hearing aids are also a frequent problem and can usually be readily corrected by an ENT technician. Hearing therapists provide more comprehensive and continuous help, both practical and psychological, by trying to help the individual make the most of residual hearing, teaching them to use every available auditory and visual clues, and also how to use their hearing aid.
- *Meals on wheels* are usually administered by local authorities and are a means of providing one hot nutritious meal a day at low cost. Disadvantages include timing, provision, quality and ethnic requirements.
- *Luncheon clubs* provide inexpensive meals, act as social centres and are mainly used by the active elderly in the immediate neighbourhood.
- *Day centres* offer a wide range of activities, cater for a mixed client group and often provide transport for the less active.

The occupational therapist (OT) role includes:

- assessment of functional level
- improving and maintaining function using graded tasks and activities to lessen fatigue and increase range of movements
- restoring function by use of craft work, remedial games
- assisting the permanently disabled to achieve maximum independence within the constraints of their disability
- the use of activities to stimulate patients mentally and physically to maintain a sense of wellbeing
- advising on appropriate aids and equipment.

Physiotherapists work closely with the occupational therapists and help patients achieve maximum independence with minimal assistance. Their role involves:

- assessment
- providing therapy to improve, maintain and/or restore function
- advising on appropriate aids and equipment.

Speech therapists are involved in:

- the assessment, treatment and management of communication disorders, including dysphasia, dysarthria, dysphonia, dyspraxia and dysfluency
- the assessment, treatment and management of swallowing disorders
- advising staff, relatives and carers about communication and swallowing.

Specialist teams exist in some areas to provide an intensive level of support to selected clients following discharge from the acute sector or following a crisis. They are designed to gradually withdraw and let the usual services take over responsibility.

Social workers work on behalf of the client in an advocacy role and enable them, through counselling, to cope with the problems of daily living and to obtain those services appropriate to their needs. They are responsible for:

- assessment of the need for independent or social services residential or nursing home
- reviewing financial ability to pay for care
- housing adaptations
- providing equipment for daily living
- day care
- day centres
- respite care in residential and nursing homes.

Activities of daily living (ADL)

These consist of the tasks undertaken daily to maintain personal care. Assessment includes ascertaining those activities that are deficient, evaluating the potential for improvement and deciding on a programme to achieve this potential.

- *Mobility*. All mobility must be considered and assessment of the environment (chairs, beds, stairs, toilet, etc.) is essential. Wheelchairs need skilled assessment to suit the needs of patients, carers and the environment.
- *Eating and drinking*. Special crockery and cutlery are available to assist the disabled person.
- *Toilet management*. This is an essential function for independence. Practical solutions such as handrails or a raised seat may be all that is required to maintain continence. Other solutions are commodes or chemical toilets, especially at night.
- *Personal hygiene and dressing*. Dressing practice and the use of aids may allow independence. Patients may require assistance, but should be encouraged to do as much as they can for themselves.
- *Communication*. Liaison with other members of the team ensures that patients with communication difficulties can receive therapy. Advice can be given on specific alarms and communication aids in the home.
- *Domestic tasks*. Training must be combined with knowledge of the patient's home circumstances and many patients perform better in their own homes than in the hospital environment. A visit to the patient's home enables assessment of the patient's ability to cope in the environment and what aids or adaptations may be necessary to facilitate this.

There are many instruments available to quantify activities of daily living (ADL), but the *Barthel Index* is the most popular and widely used in the UK. It is an ordinal scale and assesses levels of independence or dependence for 10 ADL tasks with a score of 0 (dependent) to 20 (independent).

The index is quick and easy to use and has been well validated. It can aid disability assessment and also show rehabilitation progress if repeated at intervals. The main disadvantage is that the steps on the scale are quite large and it is therefore not very sensitive to change. Also, especially for disabled people living at home, there is a marked ceiling effect in that patients can score a maximum of 20 points, but still have daily living restrictions. Extended ADL scales such as the *Nottingham ADL* score and the *Frenchay Activities Index* extend the range of the Barthel Index to include other important daily tasks such as housework, shopping and trips.

The *Barthel Index*

- Bowels
- Bladder
- Grooming
- Toilet
- Feeding
- Bed-to-chair transfers
- Walking
- dressing
- stairs
- bathing.

Assessment of mental function

Given the high prevalence of dementia and cognitive impairment in the elderly, assessment of mental function is important. This usually involves a mental test score such as the Abbreviated Mental Test Score (AMTS) or the Mini-Mental State Examination (MMSE). The AMTS is a 10-point score and tests short- and long-term memory, orientation and numeracy skills. The MMSE is a 30-point score and tests orientation, short-term memory, concentration, language and comprehension. It is important to remember that these are screening tests and not diagnostic instruments. Deafness and speech impairments can make patients appear very cognitively impaired and depressed patients often score badly. Ethnic differences and level of education achieved may also affect scores. More complex tests are available to assess higher cognitive function and are usually applied by clinical psychologists.

Abbreviated Mental Test Score (AMTS)

- Age
- Time (to nearest hour)
- Address for recall
- Year
- Where do you live (town or road)?
- Recognition of two persons
- Date of birth
- Year of start of First World War
- Name of present monarch
- Count backwards 20 to 1

Mini-Mental State Examination (MMSE)

- Orientation in time (day, date, month, year, season)
- Orientation in place (place, level, street, city/town, country)
- Registration (3 objects to repeat)
- Concentration (Serial 7s)
- Recall (the 3 objects above)
- Three-stage command
- Repeat 'no, ifs ands or buts'
- Read and obey command
- Write sentence
- Copy intersecting pentagons

9

Legal aspects

Legislation providing financial protection for the elderly

Legislation providing financial protection for the elderly with physical and mental disabilities includes the following.

Power of attorney

- Used by older person who is unable to undertake financial transactions, such as paying bills or getting money from a bank, because of physical disability.
- Person has no mental illness.
- Attorney can be a family member or a friend.

Enduring power of attorney

- Commonly used by those in early stages of dementia when they have full mental capacity to make decisions.
- Covers financial affairs only.
- Attorney has full access to financial assets of the person, including the power to write cheques.
- Once the person loses mental capacity the attorney must register this with the Court of Protection.

The Court of Protection

- Used in cases where patients lose testamentary capacity, usually as a result of dementia.
- Application can be made by an individual member of the family or through a solicitor.
- The official form requires a statement from a doctor confirming that an individual does not have testamentary capacity.

Assessment of testamentary capacity

A person is judged to have capacity to make a will if he or she:

- knows the nature of action involved in making a will
- has a reasonable grasp of the extent of their assets
- knows the person or persons to whom they are leaving their property and money
- is free of delusions, which might distort judgement.

Compulsory admission and treatment of patients with a psychiatric illness

Mental Health Act 1983

Introduction

- This Act can be used for patients with any formal mental illness, including delirium and dementia, although it is unusual to use the Act for such patients, as treatment can be given under common law in the patient's best interests.
- Treatment under the Act only applies to treatment of the mental illness itself and not to any coexisting physical illness, although it is possible to treat a physical illness which is the cause of a symptom of a mental illness.
- Although doctors have the power to recommend compulsory admission under the Act, the main right to make a formal application rests with the social worker or a relative.

Definitions included in the Act

- Mental disorder – mental illness, arrested or incomplete development of mind, psychopathic disorder and other disorder or disability of mind.
- Mental impairment – impairment of intelligence and social functioning.
- Severe mental impairment – 'a state of arrested or incomplete development of mind, which includes severe impairment of intelligence and social functioning and is associated with abnormally aggressive or seriously irresponsible conduct on the part of the person concerned'.
- Psychopathic disorder – a persistent disorder or disability of mind that results in abnormally aggressive or seriously irresponsible conduct on the part of the person concerned.
- Duties of approved social workers:
  - to gather information and co-ordinate the assessment process
  - to ensure that admission to hospital or guardianship is appropriate
  - to safeguard the civil liberties of the patient
  - to ensure that the necessary treatment recommended by the approved doctors is the least restrictive of all options.

Provisions of the Act

Section 2

- Allows formal admission to hospital for assessment, observation and subsequent treatment.
- The application can be made by the patient's relative, a social worker or a person given power to act on the patient's behalf on recommendations of two registered medical practitioners. In case of urgent need, an application can be made on a recommendation of one practitioner.
- The assessment period: 28 days.
- The grounds for application:
  - the patient is suffering from a mental disorder of a nature and degree that warrant detention for assessment (or assessment followed by treatment)
  - the detention is in the interests of the patient him or herself (health and safety) or for the protection of other people.

Section 3

- Section 3 allows admission for compulsory treatment of mental disorder or illness for six months. The grounds for application include:
  - the treatment is necessary for the health and safety of the patient and others

- the treatment is likely to alleviate or prevent deterioration of the condition
- the person has a mental illness, severe mental impairment or psychopathic disorder, the nature of which makes it appropriate to receive treatment.

- The application procedure: similar to that for sectioning under Section 2, except that under this section the nearest relative must be consulted when an applicant is a social worker.

Section 4

- Admission as an emergency by reason of 'urgent necessity' and for this only one medical recommendation is required.
- If they (social worker or relatives) cannot cope with the patient's behaviour.
- There must be an immediate significant risk to the patient or others.
- The doctor recommending emergency treatment should, if practicable, have known the patient before and have seen him in the previous 24 hours.
- The period of detention: maximum of 72 hours, but this can be converted to 28 days by seeking a second specialist opinion.
- During the first 72 hours the patient has no right of appeal.

Section 5

- This section provides holding power for a doctor or a nurse for forcibly detaining informal patients for up to six hours.
- The consultant (or deputy) can enforce the detention for 72 hours.
- This applies to patients receiving inpatient treatment for a physical condition, but not to patients being treated in the outpatient clinic or day hospital.
- Under Section 5 (2) the medical practitioner responsible for treating a patient can make an application to detain the patient in hospital by writing a report to the managers. If the medical practitioner in charge of clinical care of a patient is likely to be absent, they can nominate another in their absence.
- Under Section 5 (4) (nurse's holding power) a nurse can detain patients who are receiving treatment for mental disorder as an inpatient in a hospital if the nurse feels that it is necessary to do so for their safety or for the safety of others and it is not practicable to get a doctor to attend to the patient for the purposes of preparing the report for application. The nurse can detain the patient in hospital for six hours.

Section 7 – Guardianship

- This section allows the local authority (or a relative accepted by the local authority) to act as *guardian* to a person with a mental disorder, mental illness or mental impairment and therefore provide community care.
- It may be used where there is conflict between the wishes of the relative and what is considered to be in the best interests of the patient.
- The guardian has power:
  - to require an individual to live in a particular place
  - to require access to be given to doctors, social workers and others at any place where the individual lives
  - to attend a particular place for treatment.
- For this section effective co-operation is required: the social worker does not have the authority to remove patients from their home if they refuse to do so and this can cause major difficulties for the appointed guardian. To enforce this section, signatures of two registered practitioners (one of whom should be a specialist) are required.
- The maximum duration is six months but it is renewable for a further six months, then year to year.

Section 117

This section applies to people detained under Sections 3 and 37 of the Mental Health Act 1983. Under this, the local authority, as well as the health authority, has a duty to carry out joint assessment and provide services.

The Mental Health Commission (MHC)

The MHC has responsibility for overseeing the treatment of compulsorily detained patients and for dealing with complaints from detained people as well as their carers.

Restraint of elderly patients

- Freedom of movement is an important basic right enforceable through a writ of *babedes corpus*. The clinical use of restraint raises moral and ethical dilemmas, particularly when the individuals are too confused and therefore not competent to make a decision for themselves.
- While it is morally unjustifiable to restrain an elderly patient, there may be a case for using restraints in the case of patients who, because of their

mental condition, are at risk of harming themselves. Under these circumstances, the Act permits such an action as long as it is being performed in the best interests of the patient. (Under Section 5(4) a nurse is allowed to use the minimum force necessary to prevent a patient from leaving the hospital.)

Elderly patients who do not have acute psychiatric illness but who are considered to be at risk in their homes

National Assistance Act 1948 – Section 47

The main function of this section is to remove an individual considered to be at severe risk at home, e.g. an older person with a fractured humerus who cannot look after themselves, but who refuses to go to hospital.

Grounds for use

- A person who is suffering from a grave and chronic disease or, being aged, infirm or physically incapacitated, is living in unsanitary conditions.
- A person who is unable to look after themselves and is not receiving proper care and attention from others.

Requirement

- An order from a magistrate.
- Application usually made by a social worker on behalf of the local authority and supported by a community physician.

Patient and relatives

- Relatives have no say and the patient has a limited right of appeal.

Legislation governing provision of care and services for older people

National Assistance Act 1948 – Section 21

This Act empowers local authorities to provide accommodation for adults over 18 years of age who are:

- disabled
- ill
- in need of care as a result of age.

In 1991 the Act converted power to duty to provide temporary accommodation to:

- those who have no alternative accommodation
- those who have urgent need because they have a mental disorder or to prevent mental disorder.

National Assistance Act 1948 – Section 29

Under this section local authorities are empowered to:

- provide a social work service
- make arrangements for promoting the welfare of disabled persons (i.e. those who are deaf, blind, dumb or suffer from a mental disorder of any description or are handicapped as a result of illness, injury or other disabilities).

Chronically Sick and Disabled Persons Act 1970 – Section 2

The Act covers services such as practical assistance in the home, home adaptations, transport for a person to use services, meals and telephones.

Health Services and Public Health Act 1968 – Section 45

Under this Act, social services are empowered to provide services to older people to promote their welfare, e.g. meals, day centres, home helps, home adaptations and social work support.

The National Health Service and Community Care Act 1990

Under Section 47 of this Act the local authorities have the responsibility for planning, financing, delivery and regulation of community care services to vulnerable groups, including the elderly and mentally ill.

In most areas local social services and health services have an agreed multi-agency body that acts as an eligibility panel for persons aged 65 and over and this panel considers the community care assessment and makes a decision as to whether an individual needs:

- NHS continuing care provision for frail older people/mental health care of older people
- nursing home placement
- residential care placement
- extra care sheltered accommodation
- domiciliary/day-care packages of care requiring more than a notional maximum sum set by the local authority.

Criteria for each of the above provisions are drawn up by the local authority after full consultation with health service providers.

The Carers (Recognition and Services) Act 1995

This Act, which does not apply to Northern Ireland, enables local authorities to assess the needs of carers and individuals in need of community care services.

Caring about Carers – 1999

Published by the government to stimulate diversity and flexibility in provision of breaks for carers or direct services to carers, in order to allow respite from the direct responsibility of supervising or caring.

The Social Work (Scotland) Act 1968

Under this Act, social work departments must provide guidance, advice and assistance to people in need of care because of age, infirmity or because they have a physical illness or mental disorder.

Community Care (Delayed Discharges, etc.) Act 2003

- This act has been introduced to help achieve a sustained reduction in the number of patients who are delayed in hospital, which will also free up NHS hospital beds for other patients.
- The Act aims to:
  - improve and strengthen discharge planning
  - improve timely provision of the services patients need to transfer from one care setting to another
  - strengthen local partnership working between the health services and the SSD.
- The Act addresses:
  - communication requirements between the hospital and the SSD
  - penalties for the SSD if a delay in the patient discharge is caused by the unavailability of services.

Rights of institutionalised elderly people

All older people in an institution are by entry criteria disabled and any assessment and treatment provided must take into account their needs, their dignity and autonomy.

The National Standards Commission in line with Section 23 of the Care Standards Act 2000 (CSA) has set up standards, the aims of which are to provide measurable quality of life for older people using the services of the home.

The areas covered include the following.

Choice of home

For an individual to make a decision they must have full information about the home. The Commission therefore requires the home to produce a statement of purpose, setting out its aims and objectives, the range of facilities and services it offers, and terms and conditions. In addition it is required that:

- no older person should be admitted to a home without a full needs assessment
- the services offered by the home should be able to meet the needs identified
- an individual and their carers/relatives should be given the opportunity to visit and assess the services offered by the home.

Health and personal care

Privacy and dignity

The home's philosophy of care must ensure that residents are treated with respect and dignity and their right to privacy is respected. This should cover dying and death.

Healthcare

The home should not only promote and maintain health, but ensure access to healthcare services to meet the needs identified.

Medication

While promoting self-administration in those who are able and willing to take on this responsibility, policy and procedures should follow guidelines laid down by the Medicines Act 1968, the Royal Pharmaceutical Society (RPS), the Misuse of Drugs Act 1971 and the United Kingdom Care Commission (UKCC).

Social contact and activities

The routines of daily living and activities made available should be flexible and varied to suit and meet the expectations, preferences and capabilities of the individual, taking into account their social, religious and recreational interests.

Autonomy and choice

Individuals should be helped to exercise choice and control over their lives and this covers meals and mealtimes.

Complaints and protection

- The home should ensure that there is a clear, simple and accessible complaints procedure for use by individual residents and their relatives.
- The individual's legal rights should be protected.
- Protection from abuse/neglect – robust procedures should be in place to respond to any suspicion or evidence of abuse or neglect.

Environment

- The environment, including communal facilities, should be safe and well-maintained.
- Sufficient and suitable lavatories and washing facilities.
- Availability of specialist equipment to maximise independence, e.g. hoists, grabrails.
- Individual rooms should meet the needs of that person, e.g. a person in a wheelchair should have at least 12 square metres of usable space.
- Rooms should be furnished and equipped to assure comfort and privacy, and should meet the assessed needs of the individual. Where possible individuals should be allowed to bring in their own possessions.

Services

- All services (heating, lighting, ventilation) should meet the relevant environmental health and safety requirements and the needs of the individual.
- The home should be clean, pleasant and hygienic.

Staffing

- The skill mix of qualified/unqualified staff should be appropriate to the assessed needs of the residents.
- By 2005 there should be a minimum ratio of 50% trained members of staff (NVQ level 2 or equivalent).
- Staff training and development programme should meet National Training Organisation (NTO) workforce training targets and ensures that staff fulfil the aims of the home and meet the changing needs of the residents.

Day-to-day operations

The person in charge must be fit to be in charge, of good character and able to discharge their responsibilities fully, that is:

- qualified, competent and experienced to run a home
- have at least two years' experience in a senior management capacity
- by 2005 she should have a qualification, at level 4 NVQ
- where nursing care is provided by the home, there should be a first-level registered nurse who has a relevant management qualification.

10

Ethical issues

1 Principles of medical ethics

Four widely accepted general principles of medical ethics employed in medical decision making are:

1 *autonomy* – respecting patients' wishes and facilitating and encouraging their input into the medical decision-making process
2 *justice* – an impartial and fair approach to treatment and the distribution of resources without discrimination on the grounds of age, race, sex, religion or sexual orientation
3 *beneficence* – to do good
4 *non-maleficence* – to do no harm.

2 Consent

2i The General Medical Council proclaims that:

'Patients must be able to trust doctors with their lives and well-being . . . In particular as a doctor you must:

- treat every patient politely and considerately
- listen to patients and respect their views
- give patients information in a way they can understand
- respect the rights of patients to be fully involved in decisions about their care
- make sure that your personal beliefs do not prejudice your patients' care.'[1]

2ii The form of consent

- For a surgical procedure – written documentation or structured conversation is necessary.
- For a *trivial* intervention – patient's verbal agreement may be assumed to imply consent.

2iii When there is no valid consent

The following three approaches to surrogate decision making are helpful:

1 substituted judgement – the decision-maker, who has knowledge of prior beliefs and values of the patient, applies them to make a decision
2 best interests – involves weighing the interests an individual might have in receiving an intervention versus not receiving it
3 pure autonomy in the form of an advance directive – formulated in the form of a person's wishes in a given situation, made while competent.

2iv The law

The following outline summarises the principal elements of English consent law.[2]

- Adults have a legal right to choose whether to consent to medical treatment, to refuse it or to choose one rather than another of the treatments on offer.
- Valid consent to medical intervention provides legal defence to the health worker from civil actions in battery (unconsented touching) or negligence, and from prosecution for the crime of battery.
- For actions in battery to succeed, the plaintiff must only prove that intentional touching occurred without consent; harm need not have occurred.
- The components of a legally valid consent are broadly that the person has capacity, has been informed about the intervention and provides the consent voluntarily.
- Adults are presumed legally competent until proven otherwise.
- The legal test of competence to consent is that the individual can comprehend and retain the relevant information, believe it, weigh the information by balancing risks and benefits, and finally arrive at a choice (which need not be a rational one).
- To avoid action in battery, a health worker need only provide information relating to the nature and purpose of the health intervention.

- To avoid action in negligence, a health worker must disclose that level of information considered to be proper by a responsible body of medical opinion.
- No adult can provide a legally effective consent (or refusal) to healthcare interventions being carried out on another adult.
- Where no consent is available because the patient lacks capacity, a health worker may legally treat the patient, so long as they act in the best interests of the patient or on the basis that the treatment is immediately necessary.

3 Mental incapacity and best interests

- The right of a mentally competent adult to refuse medical or any other intervention is enshrined in UK common law and reinforced by the Human Rights Act 1998 which incorporates the European Convention on Human Rights into domestic law.
- A person may refuse treatment for reasons which are 'rational, irrational or for no reason' and a doctor may be liable in assault or battery or for breach of Article 8* of the Convention on Human Rights if he or she touches a person contrary to his or her wishes.
- If the person is mentally incapable, whether temporarily or permanently, the doctor has a duty to act in his or her best interests.
- A decision on mental capacity is ultimately a question of law for a court to decide. However, most decisions about mental capacity to make decisions about medical treatment never reach the hands of lawyers and are undertaken by the treating doctor.
- Mental incapacity is a significant issue for doctors who provide healthcare for older people because of the high prevalence of both dementia and delirium.

3i Legal rules for assessing mental capacity for medical decisions

The present legal rules for the assessment of mental capacity vary according to the decision undertaken. The rules governing capacity to make decisions about medical treatments were initially set out in 'Re C' (1994) – a case in which the High Court was asked to decide whether a schizophrenic patient from Broadmoor Hospital was mentally competent to refuse amputation of a

---

*Article 8 of the Human Rights Act is the right to private and family life, and also incorporates the right to protect the physical integrity of a person.

gangrenous leg. It was stated that an adult has the capacity to refuse medical treatment if that adult can:

1 understand and retain the information relevant to the decision in question
2 believe that information
3 weigh that information in the balance to arrive at a choice.

Although useful, it has been suggested that this test is not quite right in that a person is not necessarily mentally incapable simply because they do not believe their doctor.

'A person lacks capacity if some impairment or disturbance of mental function renders the person unable to make a decision whether to consent to or to refuse treatment. That inability will occur when:

1 the person is unable to comprehend and retain the information which is material to the decision, especially as to the likely consequences of having or not having the treatment in question
2 the person is unable to use the information and weigh it in the balance as part of the process of arriving at a decision.'

The decision about mental capacity will vary according to the gravity of the decision – the more serious the decision, the greater the capacity required.

3ii Assessing mental capacity

In cases where mental capacity is severely impaired the assessment will often be straightforward. However, where impairment is mild or moderate, the assessment may be difficult. In such cases one should make a comprehensive examination of mental function having regard to the fact that an abnormality in behaviour, language function, mood, thought, perception, insight, cognition, memory, intelligence or orientation may result in an inability to make decisions and thereby render the person mentally incapable.

Evidence from other members of the multidisciplinary team, especially nursing and therapy colleagues, and from relatives or friends may be helpful in coming to a decision.

3iii Mental capacity and the Mental Health Acts

- Mental capacity is not relevant to the working of the Mental Health Act 1983 in England and Wales and the Mental Health (Scotland) Act 1984.

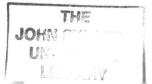

- The various sections of these Acts are not framed in terms of mental incapacity, but in terms of mental illness and the interests of the patient's health and safety and the protection of others.
- If applicable, the Acts allow the treatment of mental illness without the consent of the person.
- Although it is not possible to treat coexisting physical illness, it is possible to treat physical illness that is a cause or consequence of the mental illness. So it is possible to force-feed a patient with anorexia under the Act, whereas it is not possible to amputate a gangrenous leg simply because the patient has schizophrenia.

3iv Mental capacity for non-medical decisions

The law relating to non-medical decisions and mental incapacity is generally similar to that for medical decisions. Presently, in England and Wales, there are a variety of slightly different common-law tests for determining mental capacity relating to different decisions, i.e. there is a specific test for mental capacity to make a will, to enter into a contract, to marry, etc. The Mental Capacity Bill[3] provides one uniform test for mental capacity and a single system of law governing the way in which decisions should be made for a mentally incapable adult, whether they be related to health, social welfare or finance.

4 Confidentiality

- Confidentiality is one of the basic premises of medical practice.
- It is fundamental to a doctor–patient relationship based on trust.
- The GMC's *Duties of a Doctor*[4] states that doctors have a duty to respect the privacy of patients and to effectively protect the information given to them. This encompasses all information obtained in a professional capacity.
- The Human Rights Act 1998 also prevents health professionals from disclosing information given to them in confidence under Article 10 – the right to freedom of expression. If information is to be shared with others, then a patient's consent should always be obtained unless there are exceptional circumstances.
- But doctors have a duty of care not only to individuals but also to the rest of the community. The nature of information shared between doctors and their patients, and changes in medical practice can lead to conflicts of interest. When these occur and the question of breaching confidentiality arises, there must be clear ethical justification for doing so.

4i Sharing information with the patient's consent

- Consent must be obtained before disclosing information to another party, unless exceptional circumstances dictate otherwise. It is good practice to document this consent.
- Depending on the nature of the disclosure, this can be done formally with the patient's written consent or as a record that verbal consent has been given.
- To give consent the patient should understand the nature and effects of the disclosure and have the capacity to make the decision.
- Sharing information between health professionals to provide good healthcare is essential for good practice and therefore it is not always necessary to get explicit consent for this, provided that the patient has agreed to treatment or investigation. For instance, if a patient agrees to a specialist referral from their GP, then it is implied that they are happy for the GP to pass on details to the specialist. The specialist will, of course, receive the information in confidence.

4ii Sharing information without consent

- This can occur in an emergency situation where it is impractical, or when patients decide to withhold consent or do not have the capacity to give it. In the UK the principle of confidentiality is not considered absolute.
- The GMC offers guidance on situations when doctors may be justified in disclosing information that has been imparted to them in confidence, or when they are required to do so. These can be summarised as:
  - when it is in the best interests of the patient
  - when it is in the public interest
  - when required to by statute or law
  - for the purposes of medical research and education, or public health.
- In cases where it has not been possible to obtain consent the patient should be informed of the decision to disclose information at the earliest opportunity. Breaching confidentiality, even when justifiable, remains an infringement of patients' rights and doctors should be prepared to defend these decisions. It may be advisable to discuss the matter with a colleague or a professional body before arriving at such a decision.

4iii Legal and statutory processes

- In a court of law a judge can order the disclosure of information.
- A doctor can object if they believe the information to be irrelevant, but this decision ultimately falls to the judge.
- When lawyers or the police seek information this cannot be given without consent. The exception to this is where failure to do so would put people at risk of serious harm.
- Information must be disclosed where there is a statutory obligation to do so, for example in the notification of certain infectious diseases or in substance misuse.
- In counterbalance the Data Protection Act 1998 gives health professionals the right not to disclose information if they believe that disclosure is likely to cause serious harm to a person's physical or mental health.

4iv Medical research, education and public health

In broad terms, when information is to be used for research (audit, epidemiology), education and public health:

- information should only be given to those who are also bound by a duty of confidentiality
- consent should be sought to share information
- data should be anonymous if this will suffice.

4v Access to medical records

- Patients have a right to view their own medical records if they wish.
- Under the Data Protection Act 1998 a patient can expect to view or be supplied with a copy of their medical records.
- Information can be withheld if a doctor feels that it may be harmful to the patient or would compromise the confidentiality of others.
- In most cases the application for access to medical records is made in relation to insurance claims or employment. Information should only be imparted with the patient's written consent. It is good practice to determine whether the patient would like to see the report. Importantly, if a patient has requested non-disclosure and this is documented in the records, then the information should not be disclosed.

5 Advance directives

- An advance directive, otherwise known as a living will, is a statement of treatment preferences so as to indicate a person's wishes should the capacity for decision making be lost in the future. Based on the principle of autonomy, it aims to project this forward into possible future mental incapacity.
- For practical purposes an advance directive is normally a written document.
- In UK law, no one has the right to give consent for the treatment of another adult (the situation in Scotland is somewhat different). Faced with a patient who is unable to participate in decision making and thus unable to give consent, a doctor acts under his or her 'duty of care' in what is considered the patient's 'best interests'.
- Where conflict arises between what is being suggested by a carer or a relative and the clinician's view a decision based on the 'best interests' of the patient should be taken.
- Legally an unambiguous and informed advance directive has the same authority as a contemporaneous decision. This common-law right has been confirmed in several legal cases.

6 Issues surrounding patients' liberty to drive and the law

- In the UK, the 1988 Road Traffic Act and the more recent Motor Vehicles (Driver Licences) Regulations 1996 define severe mental disorders as a relevant disability for licensing and this includes dementia.
- The person is obliged by law to inform the DVLA about their condition. If a patient refuses to do so despite advice from their doctor and family then the doctor can inform the DVLA after informing the patient of this decision.
- Professional codes of conduct usually allow for breaking of medical confidentiality in the case of considered assessments of dangerous driving when such drivers will not cease driving.
- Courts in the UK have considered that doctors are bound to advise patients on conditions which may impair safe driving.

7 Cardiopulmonary resuscitation (CPR) and do-not-attempt-resuscitation order (DNAR)

- While CPR decisions are commonly made by hospital physicians, GPs may be involved in making such decisions if they are in charge of clinical care of patients in community hospitals.
- The new guidelines issued by professional bodies (British Medical Association (BMA), Royal College of Nursing and Resuscitation Council (UK))[5] incorporate several important changes, some of which have been included in recognition of the provisions of the Human Rights Act.
- When making the DNAR decision it is important to remember the following.
  - The goal of medicine is not to prolong life at all costs with no regard to its quality or burden of treatment on the patient.
  - A competent patient has the right to accept or refuse resuscitation after he/she has been fully informed of its benefits and risks.
  - The consultant or GP should always be prepared to discuss DNAR decisions with competent patients.
  - Under the Human Rights Act 1998 a competent patient has the right to refuse a DNAR decision made by a physician and ask them not to document it in the medical records. Under these circumstances a physician is obliged to follow this decision, provided there is a chance that resuscitation will lead to restoration of pulse and breathing.
  - In the case of an incompetent patient, the doctor should discuss the benefits and risks of CPR with close relatives/carers and other staff, and reach a decision based on what would be in the best interests of the patient. If the joint discussion reaches the conclusion that CPR would be inappropriate, as it will add nothing to the patient's wellbeing as a person, then the doctor is not required to offer it.
  - Consultants and GPs should usually consult other professionals.
  - Under the Human Rights Act, relatives and carers have a right to information with the consent of the competent patient. The role of relatives/carers is to help the doctor in decision making and to reflect what a competent patient would want in the circumstances; they do not have the right to demand or reject resuscitation or a DNAR order.
  - The overall responsibility for decisions about CPR and DNAR rests with the consultant or GP in charge of the patient's care, and this may lead to dispute with the other professionals in the multidisciplinary team.

8 Key ethical and legal issues in relation to care of older persons with dementia

- In the early stages patients with dementia have the full capacity to undertake decision making surrounding their treatment, and therefore should not be treated differently from other patients.
- Basic principles require the physician to tell the truth to the patient that he or she has dementia.
- Since there are no available preventive or therapeutic agents that can cure dementia, it is not necessary to carry out genetic testing to see if a family member has the gene or not.
- Any new effective treatment that is developed should be offered to patients; no one should be denied treatment purely on the grounds of cost.
- Patients with obvious impairment of judgement or visual–spatial difficulties should be asked to stop driving. If a person fails to take advice they should be reported to the Vehicle and Licensing Agency, even if it means breaking the rule on patient confidentiality.
- In the later stages of the disease, doctors may have to make decisions about which treatment is best for the individual. In end-stage dementia, when a person is not able to recognise loved ones, life-sustaining treatment need not be offered, but palliative care should be practised instead.
- Chemical restraints should only be used when they contribute to the safety of the patient or others, not simply for the convenience of staff.
- In the early stages of dementia, patients should be encouraged to consider enduring power of attorney, which can then be registered with the Court of Protection when the patient becomes mentally incapable.
- Patients who neglect themselves may have to be admitted to hospital under Section 47 of the National Assistance Act or moved into a residential home using Guardianship under the Mental Health Act of 1983.

9 Use of restraints in older people in hospitals, nursing homes and residential homes

1 It is important for all individuals to have freedom of movement. Therefore no one should advocate going back to the use of physical restraints of the

straitjacket type. In addition, the use of physical restraints is against the law in the UK.

2   While it is morally unjustifiable to restrain patients, especially when there are empirical research data suggesting that it is associated with ill effects, there will always be a small number of patients who, because of their agitation or tendency to wander, require restriction for their own safety.

3   In the hospital (or nursing home) setting it is essential that the hospital/ nursing home sets standards of care on use of restraints that balance the importance of the patient's freedom and requirement of the hospital or home to safeguard the patient.

4   Each individual professional advocating the use of restraint must:
    –   establish the justification for its use
    –   if possible, try to obtain consent from the proxy decision-maker for a patient who is not competent to make a decision themselves.

5   Where restraint is required as a best course of care then it may be justified without the patient's consent if the patient lacks sufficient autonomy to make any choice.

6   Law permits a hospital doctor to prescribe an injection of a tranquilliser and to summon porters to hold down a severely agitated patient while the nurse administers it, when it is for the patient's own protection.

References

1   www.gmc-uk.org/standards
2   Kennedy I and Grubb A (2000) *Medical Law: text with materials* (3e). Butterworths, London.
3   www.publications.parliament.uk
4   General Medical Council (2002) *Duties of a Doctor*. GMC, London. www.gmc-uk.org/standards/doad.htm
5   British Medical Association, Resuscitation Council (UK), Royal College of Nursing (2002) *A Joint Statement on Decisions Relating to Cardiopulmonary Resuscitation*. BMA, London.

11

Palliative care

History

- Established to improve the care of dying patients and their families.
- Focuses traditionally on patients with incurable cancer.
- Role extending to patients with non-malignant conditions.

World Health Organization definition

The World Health Organization (WHO) defines 'palliative care' as:

> An approach that improves the quality of life of patients and their families facing the problems associated with life-threatening illness, through the prevention and relief of suffering by means of early identification and impeccable assessment and treatment of pain and other problems, physical, psychological and spiritual.

Palliative care:

- provides relief from pain and other distressing symptoms
- affirms life and regards dying as a normal process
- intends neither to hasten nor postpone death
- integrates the psychological and spiritual aspects of patient care
- offers a support system to help patients live as actively as possible until death
- offers a support system to help the family cope during the patient's illness and in bereavement
- uses a team approach to address the needs of patients and their families, including bereavement counselling, if indicated
- will enhance quality of life, and may also positively influence the course of illness
- is applicable early in the course of illness, in conjunction with other therapies that prolong life, such as chemotherapy or radiation therapy,

and includes those investigations needed to better understand and manage distressing clinical complications.

Principles of a good death[1]

- To know when death is coming and to understand what can be expected.
- To be able to regain control of what happens.
- To be afforded dignity and privacy.
- To have control over pain and other symptoms.
- To have choice and control over where death occurs.
- To have access to information and expertise of whatever kind is necessary.
- To have access to any spiritual or emotional support required.
- To have access to hospital care in any location, not only in hospital.
- To have control over who is present and who shares the end.
- To be able to issue advance directives to ensure wishes are respected.
- To have time to say goodbye and control over other aspects of timing.
- To be able to leave when it is time to go and not to have life prolonged pointlessly.

Delivery of care

Palliative care was given specialist standing as recently as 1987. The multidisciplinary team approach includes the following.

- Professionals:
  - consultants in palliative medicine
  - registrars in training
  - specialist nurses
  - GPs
  - district nurses
  - occupational therapists
  - physiotherapists
  - social workers
  - dieticians
  - psychologists
  - religious leaders.
- Informal carers:
  - family
  - friends
  - neighbours
  - volunteers.

- Places of care:
  - home
  - hospital
  - hospice
  - nursing/residential homes
  - respite.

Communication between primary and secondary care is paramount – many patients spend some time at home during their terminal illness and may choose to die there.

Carers

- Relatives, friends and neighbours often become informal carers.
- Burdens may be physical, psychological, social and financial.
- Support mechanisms include:
  - provision of knowledge (diagnosis/prognosis/symptom control)
  - emergency contact
  - practical (home modifications/aids)
  - domestic
  - psychosocial including bereavement support
  - financial (carer's allowance)
  - respite (hospice/care home/day or night sitting services).

Symptom control

Pain

- Common in malignancy.
- Multiple causes (bony/visceral/neuropathic).
- Understanding of pathophysiology is crucial for effective management.
- Perception of pain is affected by depression and anxiety.
- Pain control measures include analgesic drugs, radiotherapy, anaesthetic nerve blocks, orthopaedic surgery to stabilise long bones and replace joints, transcutaneous electrical nerve stimulation (TENS), treatment of mood disorders.
- Concept of 'analgesic ladder' should be employed when prescribing analgesic drugs:
  - aspirin/paracetamol/non steroidals (mild pain)

  - codeine/dextropropoxyphene (moderate pain)
  - morphine/other opioids (severe pain)
- Consider tricyclic antidepressants and anticonvulsants for neuropathic pain and bisphosphonates for bony pain.
- Drugs should be administered on a regular basis with adequate doses available for breakthrough symptoms.
- Analgesic requirements require review every 1–2 days.
- Remember other routes of administration if oral not possible – per rectum, subcutaneous (including syringe drivers), intravenous, intramuscular.

Respiratory problems

Shortness of breath

- A manifestation of both malignant and non-malignant cardiorespiratory disease.
- Treatment depends on underlying cause (pleural or pericardial effusion/ lung metastases/pulmonary oedema/pneumonia/pulmonary embolus).
- Steroids and radiotherapy are used in stridor.
- Anxiolytics and opioids may improve distressing symptoms.
- Increases carer stress.

Cough

- Treatment should be directed at specific cause.
- Consider antitussive agents such as opioids or local anaesthetic agents.
- Hyoscine can dry up excess secretions.
- Correct positioning and physiotherapy for suction and postural drainage are helpful.

Haemoptysis

- Treatment depends on cause – tranexamic acid and radiotherapy for tumour-related bleeds and anticoagulation for pulmonary emboli.
- For major haemorrhage appropriateness of aggressive resuscitation should be reviewed – pure palliation of symptoms with analgesics and sedatives may be preferable.

Gastrointestinal complaints

Nutritional status

- Anorexia is common.
- Weight loss is a poor prognostic indicator.
- Cachexia is associated with reduced caloric intake, malabsorption and metabolic abnormalities including release of cytokines in malignancy.
- Therapeutic options include nutritional supplementation and appetite stimulants.

Mouth care

- Commonly neglected.
- Oral cavity should be reviewed on a daily basis.
- Twice-daily brushing of teeth/dentures and tongue advised for comfort as well as hygiene.
- Soothe dry lips with petroleum jelly.
- Maintain adequate hydration.
- Antifungal agents such as topical nystatin or oral preparations, e.g. fluconazole, should be used to treat candidiasis.
- Topical anaesthetic agents ease the pain of a sore mouth.
- Consider topical steroids/antibiotics for aphthous ulcers.

Nausea and vomiting

- Culprits include drugs, hypercalcaemia, uraemia, gastric inflammation/ ulceration/stasis and constipation and/or bowel obstruction.
- Treatment should be directed at underlying cause.
- Antiemetics can provide symptomatic relief – mode of action is important:
  - anticholinergics, e.g. hyoscine
  - antihistamines, e.g. cyclizine
  - butyrophenones, e.g. haloperidol
  - phenothiazines, e.g. methotrimeprazine
  - prokinetics, e.g. domperidone, metoclopramide
  - 5HT receptor blockers, e.g. ondansetron.

Bowel problems

- Constipation is a common consequence of malignancy and may be caused by:
  - drugs, e.g. opioids, anticholinergics
  - tumour, e.g. hypercalcaemia, spinal cord compression, abdominopelvic disease
  - general, e.g. immobility, dehydration, inaccessible toilet facilities.
- A combination of oral and rectal laxatives may be required.
- Elderly patients with non-malignant disease are prone to constipation with faecal impaction and overflow diarrhoea.
- Diarrhoea in patients with cancer is less common than constipation and may be related to drugs (e.g. laxatives, chemotherapy), radiotherapy, malabsorption and bowel obstruction.
- Treatment of diarrhoea should be directed at underlying cause and may necessitate use of codeine or loperamide.

Skin care

- Terminally ill patients are at high risk of developing pressure sores.
- Common sites include heels, ankles, knees, buttocks, spine, elbows and shoulder blades.
- Predisposing factors include immobility, malnutrition, confusion, incontinence, pain, inappropriate mattresses and inadequately trained carers.
- Pressure areas require daily review.
- Risk assessment scores, e.g. Waterlow, help identify high-risk patients.
- See Chapter 15 for management details.

Psychiatric problems

Delirium

- Elderly patients are particularly at risk in view of impairments of hearing, vision and cognition.
- Other predisposing factors: drugs including polypharmacy, electrolyte abnormalities, hypercalcaemia, sepsis.
- Underlying cause should be treated (sedatives may be required in some cases).

Anxiety and depression

- May affect both patients and carers.
- Effects can be physical as well as psychological.
- Consider psychology/psychiatry review +/– drug therapy.

Medical emergencies

Hypercalcaemia

- Bisphosphonate therapy for symptomatic patients and when calcium >3 mmol/l. Monthly infusions may be required to maintain normo-calcaemia.

Spinal cord compression

- MRI is the investigation of choice.
- Treatment options include steroids, radiotherapy and/or surgery in suitable patients.

Pathological fracture

- Prophylactic internal fixation in selected cases.
- Radiotherapy may halt progression of bony metastases.

Superior vena caval obstruction

- Mainstay treatments are steroids and radiotherapy.

Non-malignant conditions

Traditionally, palliative care has specialised in the care of patients with incurable cancer. Provision of services should, however, be on the basis of need rather than diagnosis. Other patient groups that could benefit from a palliative approach include those with chronic neurological disorders and cardio-respiratory disease. Justification for palliative care for heart failure includes:

- incidence 1–2%
- worse prognosis than some forms of cancer

- psychological and social morbidity

Specialist heart failure nurses could aid symptom control, reduce hospital admission rates and provide psychological support.

Ethical issues at the end of life

Power of attorney

A patient can grant durable power of attorney to someone trusted so that they can make decisions regarding their healthcare, should there come a time when the patient is no longer able to express their wishes.

Advance directives

- A competent patient has the right to refuse medical treatment.
- Written declarations of refusal are called advance directives or 'living wills'.

Euthanasia

- Active voluntary euthanasia (assisted suicide), where a doctor ends a patient's life at their request, is against the law in the UK.
- Using high doses of opiates to ease suffering may cause death (passive euthanasia), but is legal due to good intent (double-effect principle).

Withholding/withdrawing life-prolonging treatment

- High levels of carer anxiety often surround this issue.
- There is no evidence that artificial hydration or nutrition influence survival or symptom control in dying patients – drips and nasogastric tubes could be classed as unnecessary intrusions.

Cardiopulmonary resuscitation (CPR)

- CPR is inappropriate if:
  - there is virtually no chance of re-establishing cardiac output
  - successful resuscitation would result in a quality of life unacceptable to the patient
  - it is contrary to the competent patient's expressed wishes.
- Discussing CPR issues with palliative patients in whom resuscitation is deemed to be futile should be avoided.

Bereavement

- Shock leads to despair and eventually to adjustment.
- Support services are available.

Ethnic minority groups

- The UK is a multicultural society.
- Views of death and dying vary considerably between cultures.
- Religious needs should be respected.
- Healthcare professionals require training in transcultural medicine.

Pathway for elderly patients requiring terminal care in hospital

Developed at St Pancras Hospital in 2000.

This checklist should be completed on at least a once-weekly basis for patients who are deemed to have a prognosis of four weeks or less by the multidisciplinary team. Please circle yes or no for each question. If the response is 'no', document why.

Patient's name: DOB:

Name of member of staff completing form:

1 Life-prolonging treatment
CPR status   Date

Has a DNR order been:

- documented?   Y   N
- discussed with family/carers?   Y   N
- discussed with patient?   Y   N

Artificial hydration/nutrition   Date

Have decisions regarding the use of intravenous fluids and nasogastric feeding been:

- documented?   Y   N
- discussed with family/carers?   Y   N
- discussed with patient?   Y   N

Antibiotic therapy   Date

Has the use of antibiotics in the face of life-threatening sepsis been:

- documented?   Y   N
- discussed with family/carers?   Y   N
- discussed with patient?   Y   N

Inappropriate investigations   Date

Has it been documented that the patient should not be subjected to unnecessary investigations such as blood tests and x-rays?   Y   N

Advance directives   Date

Has the patient made a 'living will'?   Y   N
If so, have the patient's wishes been fulfilled?   Y   N

General management   Date

Are all staff involved with the care of the patient aware of the above decisions?   Y   N

2 Symptom control   Date

Has control of the following symptoms been addressed?

- pain   Y   N
- agitation/restlessness   Y   N
- confusion   Y   N
- anxiety/depression   Y   N
- insomnia   Y   N
- dysphagia   Y   N
- nausea/vomiting   Y   N
- constipation/diarrhoea   Y   N
- dry/sore mouth   Y   N

● shortness of breath	Y	N
● cough	Y	N
● noisy breathing	Y	N
● urinary incontinence/retention	Y	N
● pressure sores	Y	N
● seizures	Y	N

Do the nursing staff know what action to take should these symptoms develop, especially during on-call periods?   Y   N

Is medication prescribed for symptom control (regular/PRN)? Y   N

Is medication delivered by an appropriate route?   Y   N

Has unnecessary medication been discontinued?   Y   N

Has the patient been reviewed by the palliative care team?   Y   N

3 Place of care   **Date**

Has the patient's desired place of care been discussed?   Y   N

Is transfer to another place of care considered appropriate by the patient (e.g. hospice/readmission from home)?   Y   N

Are you aware of the patient's religious/cultural/spiritual needs and have they been met?   Y   N

4 Family/carers   **Date**

Have the religious/cultural/spiritual needs of family members/carers been addressed?   Y   N

Has discussion taken place with regard to the patient's desired place of care?   Y   N

Are the family willing to care for the patient at home if so desired by the patient?   Y   N

Are the family capable of providing that care?   Y   N

If the patient returns home, have the family been counselled as to the management of crises?   Y   N

If the patient is to return home to die, has the GP been informed?
                                                                        Y   N

Reference

1   Debate of the Age Health and Care Study Group (1999) *The Future of Health and Care of Older People: the best is yet to come.* Age Concern, London.

Part III

Clinical problems encountered in old age

12

Falls

Definition

An event which results in a person coming to rest unintentionally on the ground or other lower level, not as a result of a major intrinsic event such as a stroke or overwhelming hazard. (*Tinetti et al*. 1988)[1]

Classification

- **Faller** – someone who has fallen at least once in a given time period, e.g. 6–12 months.
- **Recurrent faller** – someone who has fallen twice or more during a defined time.
- **Once-only faller** – closely related to non-fallers.

Statistics

- A major cause of disability.
- The leading cause of mortality due to injury in older people over 75 years in the UK.
- 35–40% of community-dwelling people aged over 65 years fall annually
- Rates are higher in those aged over 75 years.
- Incidence rates for nursing home residents and hospital inpatients are almost three times greater.
- 50% of fallers do so repeatedly.
- For previous fallers, the risk of falling again in the subsequent year is increased by two thirds.
- The majority of falls occur in the usual place of residence – in the home, the bedroom, kitchen and dining room are the most common settings.

- Indoor falls are associated with frailty, whereas outdoor events are more likely to occur in more active people.
- People aged under 75 years are more likely to fall outdoors than those older than 75.
- 80% of falls in the community occur during the day as opposed to at night.
- 40–60% of falls lead to injuries.
- Overall, injury rates are higher in institutionalised patients.

Risk factors

- More than 400 risk factors for falling have been identified.
- There is often a multifactorial aetiology.
- The five major categories cover the following:
  1 Environmental
     - loose carpets and rugs
     - steep stairs
     - poor lighting
     - slippery floors
     - poorly fitting footwear and clothes
     - lack of safety equipment, e.g. grabrails
     - inaccessible lights or windows.
  2 Drugs
     - alcohol
     - analgesics
     - antiarrhythmics
     - antidepressants
     - antihistamines
     - antihypertensives
     - antipsychotics
     - sedatives
     - polypharmacy (more than four drugs).
  3 Medical conditions
     - arthritis
     - cognitive impairment
     - depression
     - parkinsonism
     - postural hypotension
     - previous falls
     - stroke
     - visual impairment.

4 Nutritional factors
   –   calcium and vitamin D deficiency.
5 Lack of exercise.

Consequences

Injury

- 40–60% of falls lead to injury
- 30–50% are minor
- 5–6% are major (excluding fracture)
- 5% result in fracture.

Hospital admission

Admission rates due to falls are six times higher in people aged over 85 years compared to those in the 65–69-year-old age group.

Psychological

- A third of those aged over 60 years develop a fear of falling.
- Loss of confidence.
- Post-fall anxiety.
- Self-imposed functional limitation.
- Social isolation.
- Depression.

Disability

- Subsequent dependency.

Long lie

- Hypothermia.
- Pressure sores.
- Dehydration.

- Rhabdomyolysis.
- Bronchopneumonia.

Institutionalisation

Fall-related accidents are predisposing factors in 40% of events leading to long-term care in older people.

National Service Framework for Older People: Standard 6: Falls (2001)[2]

Aims

- To reduce the number of falls that result in serious injury.
- To ensure effective treatment and rehabilitation.
- To provide advice on prevention through a specialised falls service.

Prevention

Population approach

- Public health strategies:
  - physical activity
  - healthy eating
  - reduced smoking.
- Environmental strategies:
  - clear pavements
  - street lighting.
- Information provision:
  - leaflets.

Individual approach

- Targeting risk factors.

Specialised falls service

Older people who fall should be referred if any of the following apply:

- previous fragility fracture
- emergency department attendance with a fall
- ambulance called after a fall
- two or more intrinsic risk factors and a fall
- frequent unexplained falls
- unsafe housing conditions
- fear of falling.

Intervention

- Diagnosis and treatment of medical problems.
- Physiotherapy and occupational therapy assessment.
- Equipment to improve home safety.
- Social care support.

Rehabilitation

The aims of rehabilitation are to:

- improve stability during standing, transferring and walking through
  - balance training
  - muscle strengthening
  - improving flexibility
  - providing appropriate safety equipment
- regain independence and confidence
- modify the home environment and remove hazards
- teach strategies to cope with further falls
- establish a network of community support if required.

Long-term support

- Pendant alarms.
- Personal or domestic services.
- Social activities.
- Monitoring of needs.

Falls service

- By April 2005 all hospital trusts should have an established falls service.
- Local policies for referral should be developed.
- Members of the team should include:
  - consultants in geriatrics
  - nurses
  - physiotherapists
  - occupational therapists
  - social workers
  - pharmacists
  - podiatrists.
- Access to the following professionals should be available:
  - dieticians
  - optometrists
  - orthotists
  - ophthalmologists
  - audiologists
  - translators.
- *See* Figure 12.1 Falls care pathway.

Hip protectors

- Advocated as a means of reducing the risk of hip fracture following a fall.
- Reduce the force transmitted to the proximal femur through the greater trochanter.
- Two types: energy-absorbing padding; semi-rigid plastic shield.
- Should be used at all times when at risk of falling (including at night).
- Problems with adherence especially in community settings (uncomfortable/unsightly/difficult to get on and off).
- Cost £40 a pair (each user ideally needs 3 pairs).
- Evidence suggests that hip protectors can reduce the incidence of hip fracture in high risk elderly people in institutional care and in highly motivated community dwellers.

References

1 Tinetti ME, Speechley M and Ginter SF (1988) Risk factors for falls among elderly persons living in the community. *N Engl J Med.* **319**: 1701–7.
2 Department of Health (2001) National Service Framework for Older People. DoH, London.

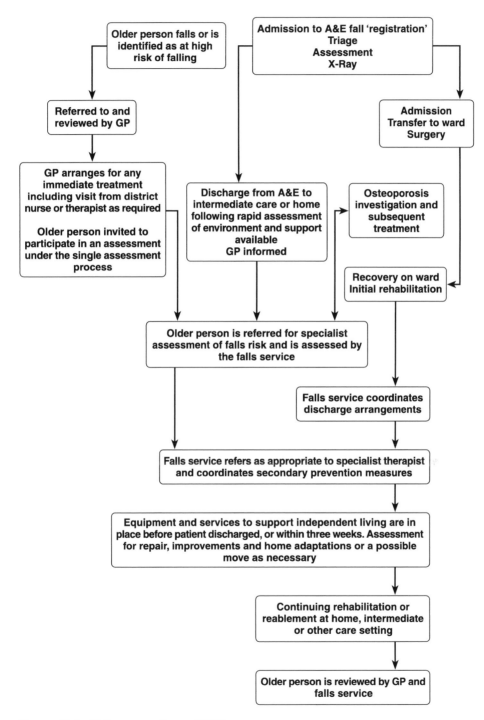

Figure 12.1   Falls care pathway (NSF).

13

Osteoporosis

Osteoporosis can be defined as:

> A progressive systemic skeletal disease characterised by low bone mass and microarchitectural deterioration of bone tissue with a consequent increase in bone fragility and susceptibility to fracture.[1]

> Bone with a density below the mean value for a young adult by >2.5 standard deviations as determined by DEXA scanning.[1]

Pathology

Three types of cells are involved in the continuous process of bone remodelling:

- osteoclasts: resorb bone
- osteoblasts: synthesise bone matrix
- osteocytes: mature osteoblasts that maintain extracellular components of bone.

Bone loss occurs if resorption exceeds formation. Peak bone mass is attained by 30 years of age.

Statistics

- 1 in 3 women and 1 in 12 men sustain osteoporotic fractures.
- Over 200 000 osteoporotic fractures are diagnosed in the UK each year.
- Spine, hip and forearm are the most commonly affected sites.
- Other sites include proximal humerus, pelvis and lower limb.
- Hip fractures alone account for over 20% of orthopaedic bed occupancy.

- Overall annual cost to the NHS is over £940m (likely to rise as population ages).
- Devastating consequences of hip fracture:[3]
  - 20% 12-month mortality
  - 50% fail to return to independent living at one year
  - 40% are unable to walk independently
  - 60% have difficulty with at least one essential ADL
  - 80% are restricted in other activities, e.g. driving, shopping
  - 27% enter a nursing home for the first time.
- Osteoporosis remains underdetected and undertreated in the elderly.

Risk factors

- Untreated hypogonadism (premature menopause/secondary amenorrhoea/primary hypogonadism in women, primary or secondary hypogonadism in men).
- Glucocorticoid therapy (7.5 mg/day >6 months).
- Other drugs (e.g. anticonvulsants/heparin/lithium/thyroxine over-replacement).
- Chronic disease (e.g. hyperparathyroidism/hyperthyroidism/liver disease).
- Radiological osteopenia.
- Family history.
- Reduced calcium and vitamin D intake.
- Smoking.
- Excess alcohol.
- Prolonged immobility.
- Caucasian.
- Additional risk factors for fracture:
  - previous fragility fracture
  - recurrent falls
  - low body mass index.

Clinical features

- Usually asymptomatic until fractures occur.
- Back pain secondary to vertebral crush fractures.
- Thoracic kyphosis resulting in loss of height.

Investigation

- If clinically indicated, organise appropriate simple tests to exclude other pathology, e.g.:
  - myeloma (FBC/ESR/serum electrophoresis/urinary Bence Jones protein)
  - bony metastases (calcium/LFTs)
  - spinal x-rays may reveal lytic/sclerotic lesions.
- Premenopausal women and men with osteoporosis should undergo specialist assessment to determine cause.
- Consider DEXA scanning.

Dual energy x-ray absorptiometry (DEXA)

- High specificity but low sensitivity for predicting future fracture risk.
- Not suitable as a population screening tool.
- Royal College of Physicians' guidelines recommend DEXA in the presence of strong risk factors.
- Useful in monitoring bone loss, assessing effect of treatment and avoiding inappropriate therapy.

Clinical guidelines for the prevention and treatment of osteoporosis: Royal College of Physicians (2000)[2]

A fragility fracture (from standing height or less/prevalent vertebral deformity) is a strong independent risk factor for further fracture and may be regarded as an indication for treatment without the need for bone mineral density measurement when the clinical history is unequivocal.

Pharmacological interventions

Bisphosphonates

- Licensed for prevention and treatment in postmenopausal women and glucocorticoid-induced osteoporosis.
- Inhibit activation and function of osteoclasts.
- May directly stimulate formation of bone by osteoblasts.

- Poor oral absorption requires them to be taken on an empty stomach with a glass of water, the patient remaining upright for 30 minutes to reduce risk of oesophageal irritation.
- Side-effects include oesophageal ulceration/stricture, constipation and renal impairment.
- Optimum duration of use unclear.

Alendronate

- Prevention – 5 mg daily.
- Treatment – 10 mg daily or 70 mg weekly.

Risedronate

- Prevention and treatment – 5 mg daily.

Etidronate

- 400 mg daily for 14 days then calcium carbonate; 500 mg daily for 76 days for prevention and treatment.
- May be more beneficial than alendronate and risedronate for vertebral osteoporosis.

Calcitonin

- Licensed for prevention and treatment of postmenopausal osteoporosis.
- Natural hormone secreted by the parathyroid gland.
- Inhibits osteoclast function.
- 100 IU plus calcium 600 mg/vitamin D 400 IU daily.
- Parenteral only.
- Side-effects: nausea, vomiting, diarrhoea and flushing.
- Less effective than bisphosphonates.

Hormone replacement therapy

Recent trial data on HRT have led the Committee on Safety of Medicines to strongly recommend that it no longer be used as first-line choice in prevention and treatment of osteoporosis – unless menopausal symptoms are intolerable an alternative agent should be used.

Raloxifene

- Licensed for prevention and treatment of postmenopausal osteoporosis.
- A selective estrogen receptor modulator.
- 60 mg daily.
- Potential side-effects include hot flushes, leg oedema and thrombo-embolism.
- Has not yet demonstrated reduced fracture incidence at all the major sites.

Calcium and vitamin D

- Licensed for prevention of hip and non-vertebral fractures.
- Especially useful in frail, housebound elderly and residential/nursing home residents.
- For example, Calcichew D3 forte 2 tablets daily.

Calcitriol

- Licensed for treatment of postmenopausal osteoporosis.
- A metabolite of vitamin D.
- 0.25 mg daily.

Grades of evidence of anti-fracture efficacy of pharmacological interventions in postmenopausal women

	Spine	Non-vertebral	Hip
Alendronate	A	A	A
Risedronate	A	A	A
Etidronate	A	B	B
Calcitonin	A	B	B
HRT	A	A	B
Raloxifene	A	nd	nd
Calcium/Vitamin D	nd	B	B
Calcitriol	A	A	nd

Grade A: meta-analysis of randomised controlled trials or at least one RCT or at least one well-designed controlled study without randomisation

Grade B: at least one other type of well-designed quasi-experimental study or well-designed non-experimental descriptive study

Grade C: from expert committee reports/opinions and/or clinical experience of authorities

nd: not demonstrated

Lifestyle advice

- Adequate dietary intake of calcium and vitamin D.
- Regular weight-bearing exercise.
- Avoidance of alcohol and tobacco.

Hip protectors

See Chapter 12 on Falls.

Surgery

Prompt surgical treatment and adequate postoperative rehabilitation should be available.

Osteoporosis in men

- The WHO definition of osteoporosis as bone mineral density >2.5 standard deviations below the mean value for young adults has only been established for women.
- As there is no established treatment for men, referral to a specialist centre is advised for investigation of underlying causes.

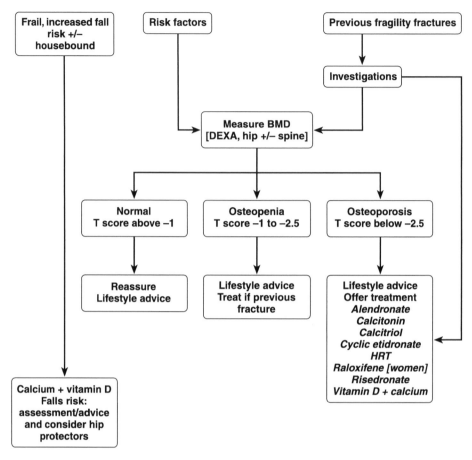

Figure 13.1 Osteoporosis – an algorithm for management.[1]

National Service Framework for older people

Osteoporosis is a target area for improvement in Standard 6 of the NSF: Falls (*see* Chapter 12 on falls).

Roles of the geriatrician in the management of osteoporosis and fractures in the elderly

- Dissemination of information into the primary care sector with regard to calcium and vitamin D prescriptions for frail, housebound elderly people and residents of care homes, and the encouragement of weight-bearing exercise if possible.

- Development of local policies for the optimal management and follow-up of older patients presenting to the emergency department with falls and/ or fracture.
- Development of an inpatient orthogeriatric service encompassing:
  - optimisation of preoperative care
  - prevention/management of postoperative complications
  - falls risk factor identification
  - secondary prevention of fracture
  - co-ordination of multidisciplinary rehabilitation
  - discharge planning
  - ensuring appropriate follow-up arrangements.

References

1 World Health Organization (1994) *Assessment of Fracture Risk and its Application to Screening for Postmenopausal Osteoporosis: Report of the World Health Organization Study Group.* WHO Technical Report Series No. 843. World Health Organization, Geneva.
2 Royal College of Physicians and Bone and Tooth Society of Great Britain (2000) *Osteoporosis: clinical guidelines for prevention and treatment.* Update on pharmacological interventions and an algorithm for management. www.rcplondon.ac.uk.pubs.wp_osteo_update.htm
3 Cooper C (1997) The crippling consequences of fractures and their impact on quality of life. *Am J Med.* **103**: 125–75.

14

Mental health problems

General

- Common in the elderly population.
- Important conditions include:
  - dementia
  - delirium
  - depression
  - anxiety
  - sleep disturbance
  - chronic schizophrenia.

National Service Framework for Older People: Standard 7 – Mental Health (2001)

Aims

- To promote good mental health in older people.
- To ensure early diagnosis.
- To provide access to specialist care and an integrated approach to assessment and treatment.
- To support carers.

Dementia

Definition

Dementia is a term used to describe a group of illnesses in which there is progressive impairment of memory and other cognitive function.

Main types of dementia in the older population

- Alzheimer's disease (60% of cases).
- Vascular dementia (20% of cases).
- Dementia with Lewy bodies (15% of cases).

Statistics

- 600 000 people in the UK have dementia.
- Prevalence increases with age:
  - 5% of >65s
  - 20% of >80s.
- Estimated number of cases by 2026: 840 000; by 2050: 1.2 million.

Clinical features

- Cognitive function:
  - progressive loss of short-term memory
  - difficulty in registration and recall of new information
  - language problems, e.g. repetition.
- Behavioural changes:
  - aggression, disinhibition, social withdrawal, wandering, disorientation
  - inability to perform usual activities of daily living.
- Psychiatric problems:
  - associated mood disorder
  - delusions/hallucinations.
- Physical debility:
  - self-neglect
  - incontinence
  - falls.

Diagnosis

Collateral history

- Patient's account may be unreliable.
- Background information from relatives, friends, neighbours and health professionals can be invaluable.
- Assists with diagnosis.
- Highlights problems that may be encountered on a day-to-day basis, e.g. difficulties with personal care, domestic tasks, self-administration of medication, attendance at medical appointments, use of public transport and financial issues.

Assessment of cognitive function (see pp. 52, 53)

- Abbreviated Mental Test Score (AMTS) (*see* p. 53).
- Mini-Mental State Examination (MMSE) (*see* p. 53).
- Used in conjunction with other methods of assessment, these tests can assist in the diagnosis.
- *MMSE* *Degree of cognitive impairment*

  22–26   mild
  10–21   moderate
   0–9   severe

Clinical examination

- May elicit clues to diagnosis, e.g. self-neglect.
- Important to exclude other pathology as a cause for symptoms.

Investigation

Certain cases may warrant further tests, e.g. blood tests (full blood count, renal/liver/thyroid function tests, calcium, vitamin B12, folate), CT brain.

Management

Non-pharmacological

- Psychological interventions include cognitive, behavioural and emotion-focused approaches.
- Assistance with activities of daily living.
- Reduction of carer burden through education and support.

Pharmacological

- Patients exhibiting extreme behavioural problems may require small doses of sedative medication, e.g. haloperidol, lorazepam.
- Cholinesterase inhibitors are licensed for use in mild/moderate Alzheimer's disease (AD).
- Memantine (NMDA antagonist) can be used in more severe cases of AD.

Memory clinics

- Provide a multidisciplinary specialist service.
- May be run by psychogeriatricians, consultants in care of the elderly or neurologists.
- Aims are to assess and treat cognitive and behavioural symptoms, monitor response to therapy, slow progression of disease and provide information/support to carers.
- National Service Framework suggests that patients should be referred for specialist advice early and particularly in certain instances:
  - uncertain diagnosis
  - difficult behavioural or psychological symptoms
  - safety concerns
  - risk of abuse or self-harm
  - determination of mental capacity.

Carers

- Family members, friends or neighbours often take on the role of informal carer when an elderly person develops dementia.
- Pressures may be emotional, social, financial and physical.

- Respite should be offered in the form of day-centre care, sitter services and either short- or long-term admission to a convalescence facility or psycho-geriatric ward.
- Charitable organisations such as the Alzheimer's Disease Society can provide information and support for carers.

Alzheimer's disease

- Commonest form of dementia in the older population.
- Affects 15 million people worldwide.
- Direct cost to NHS per year is approximately £1 billion.
- A neurodegenerative disease associated with characteristic pathological changes in neocortex and hippocampus:
  - neurofibrillary tangles (containing tau protein)
  - senile plaques (with extracellular deposits of beta-amyloid)
  - loss of neurones and neuronal synapses (including loss of cholinergic transmission).
- Aetiology remains unknown.

Clinical features (Diagnostic and Statistical Manual of Mental Disorders)

A   Development of multiple cognitive deficits manifested by both:

1   memory impairment (impaired ability to learn new information or to recall previously learned information)
2   one (or more) of the following cognitive disturbances:
   - aphasia (language disturbance)
   - apraxia (impaired ability to carry out motor activities despite intact motor function)
   - agnosia (failure to recognise or identify objects despite intact sensory function)
   - disturbance in executive functioning (planning, organisation).

B   Cognitive deficits in A1 and A2 each cause significant impairment in social or occupational functioning and represent a significant decline from a previous level of functioning.

C Course characterised by gradual onset and continuing cognitive decline.

D Cognitive deficits in A1 and A2 are not due to any of the following:
  – other central nervous conditions that cause progressive deficits in memory and cognition (e.g. cerebrovascular disease, Parkinson's disease, Huntington's chorea, subdural haematoma, normal pressure hydrocephalus, tumour)
  – systemic conditions that are known to cause dementia (e.g. hypothyroidism, deficiencies in vitamin B12/folate/niacin, hypercalcaemia, neurosyphilis and HIV)
  – substance-induced conditions.

E Deficits do not occur exclusively during the course of the delirium.

F Disturbance is not better accounted for by another disorder, e.g. depression.

Drug therapy in Alzheimer's disease

Cholinesterase inhibitors

- Alzheimer's disease is characterised by a cholinergic deficit.
- Cholinesterase inhibitors enhance cholinergic neurotransmission by delaying breakdown of acetylcholine.
- Three drugs (donepezil, galantamine and rivastigmine) are licensed in the UK for use in mild/moderate AD.
- Patients should be on the highest tolerable dose for maximal effect.
- It may be worthwhile switching to a different agent when the first begins to lose effect.
- Side-effects include gastrointestinal upset, headache, dizziness, fatigue, syncope and bradycardias.
- Current UK prescribing distribution:
  – donepezil   70%
  – galantamine   18%
  – rivastigmine   12%
- Drug costs are approximately £42 million/year (may be offset by delay in admissions to residential/nursing care facilities).
- NICE Guidance (2001):[2]
  – cognition, global/behavioural functioning and activities of daily living must be assessed before prescription
  – MMSE score must be ≥ 12
  – compliance must be assured

- – drug should only be continued if, at 2–4 months, specialist assessment shows improvement or no deterioration in MMSE score, or there is evidence of improvement based on behavioural or functional assessment
- – patients should be reviewed every six months and treatment only continued while MMSE remains ≥ 12
- – not currently licensed for use in other forms of dementia or more severe cases of AD, but results of trials are awaited.

Memantine

- Excessive activation of the NMDA (N-methyl-D-aspartate) receptor by glutamate (an excitatory amino acid) may contribute to destruction of cholinergic neurones.
- Memantine is an NMDA receptor antagonist.
- Licensed for use in moderate/severe AD in the UK since 2002.
- May stabilise symptoms.
- Optimum dose 20 mg/day.
- Potential side-effects include confusion, hallucinations, dizziness, headaches and fatigue.
- Trials under way to assess efficacy in other dementia types.

Vascular dementia

- Second most common form of dementia.
- Characterised by abrupt onset and stepwise deterioration.
- Certain abilities may remain unaffected depending on areas of brain involved.
- Risk factors include:
  - – stroke
  - – transient ischaemic attacks (TIA)
  - – atrial fibrillation
  - – hypertension
  - – diabetes mellitus
  - – smoking
  - – hypercholesterolaemia
  - – family history of vascular disease.
- CT brain will show evidence of ischaemic damage.
- Primary prevention is important in high-risk groups.
- Secondary prevention is paramount in reducing the chance of further events.

Dementia with Lewy bodies

- Microscopic deposits (Lewy bodies) cause damage to nerve cells.
- Characterised by parkinsonism, visual hallucinations and falls in addition to progressive cognitive impairment.

Delirium

Definition

Delirium is a syndrome characterised by concurrent disturbance of consciousness and attention, perception, thinking, memory, psychomotor behaviour, emotion and the sleep–wake cycle.[3]

Statistics

- Up to 30% of medical inpatients are affected.
- Increases morbidity and mortality rates, length of hospital stay and rate of institutionalisation.

Predisposing factors

- Dementia.
- Acute illness.
- Sensory impairment (vision/hearing).
- Medication.
- Change of environment (often in association with pre-existing dementia).

Causes

- Infection, e.g. urine, chest.
- Drugs, e.g. antibiotics, anticholinergics, anticonvulsants, anti-parkinsonian drugs, opiate analgesics, psychotropics, steroids.
- Drug withdrawal, e.g. alcohol, benzodiazepines.
- Metabolic, e.g. electrolyte disturbances, dehydration, hepatic dysfunction, hyper/hypoglycaemia, hyper/hypothyroidism, hypoxia.

- Neurological, e.g. stroke, transient ischaemic attacks, post-ictal, space-occupying lesions, meningitis, encephalitis.

Clinical features

- Acute onset (hours/days).
- Fluctuating intensity.
- Impaired consciousness.
- Disorientation in time, place and person.
- Poor attention.
- Visual hallucinations.
- Some patients become withdrawn ('quiet delirium').
- Most recover within four weeks but symptoms may last up to six months.

Complications

- Falls and subsequent injury.
- Consequences of medication non-compliance.
- Loss of functional independence.
- Incontinence.
- Inadequate nutrition.
- Dehydration.
- Oversedation.
- Pressure sores in hypoactive cases.

Assessment

- Investigations to consider include routine blood tests, urinalysis and CT brain.
- Diagnostic scale, e.g. CAM – Confusion Assessment Method*:[4]
  - Feature 1: acute onset and fluctuating course
  - Feature 2: inattention
  - Feature 3: disorganised thinking
  - Feature 4: altered level of consciousness.

*Diagnosis by this method requires presence of features 1 and 2 and either feature 3 or 4.

Management

Non-drug strategies

- Nurse in a safe area, preferably a side room, with adequate lighting and low noise levels.
- Avoid inter/intra-ward transfers.
- Maintain continuity of nursing staff if possible.
- Reassure and talk calmly.
- Ensure provision of glasses and hearing aids.
- Provide clocks to assist orientation and familiar objects.
- Explain situation to visitors and encourage their support.
- Avoid physical restraints.

Medication

- Sedation may need to be considered in some cases:
  - risk of self-harm or injury to others
  - severe agitation
  - essential investigations or treatment required.
- Low doses of antipsychotics (e.g. haloperidol) or benzodiazepines (e.g. lorazepam) can be used.

Depression

Statistics

- Most common psychiatric disorder in over-65s (affects 10–15%).
- 3–5% over 65 years have severe depression.
- Associated with high suicide rate.
- Increases morbidity and mortality.

Precipitating factors

- Bereavement.
- Retirement.
- Change in living circumstances, e.g. institutionalisation.
- Poor health (twice as many people with chronic illnesses have depression compared to the physically well).

- Disability.
- Social isolation.
- Past history of depression.
- Family history of mood disorder.
- Certain drugs, e.g. methyl dopa, beta-blockers, neuroleptics, steroids, opiates and alcohol.

Clinical features

- Low mood.
- Anhedonia.
- Sleep disturbance (early morning wakening).
- Fatigue.
- Poor memory and concentration.
- Agitation.
- Feelings of guilt, helplessness or hopelessness.
- Loss of appetite and weight.
- Preoccupation with death.
- Suicidal thoughts.
- Delusions.
- Somatic symptoms with no identifiable physical cause.

Risk factors for suicide

- Male.
- Previous suicidal attempt.
- Bereavement.
- Painful medical conditions.
- Social isolation.
- Alcohol dependence.

Diagnosis

- May be difficult to diagnose in older people:
  - patients may minimise their feelings of sadness
  - presentation with physical complaints is common
  - concomitant illness may challenge assessment.

- Geriatric Depression Scale-30 is a 30-point questionnaire assessing mainly cognitive aspects rather than physical symptoms: scores greater than 11 are significant.
- Assess suicide risk.
- Identify any precipitants.
- Exclude physical causes of low mood, e.g. hypothyroidism.
- Differential diagnoses include anxiety, grief and dementia.

Management

Psychological therapies

Cognitive behavioural therapy, interpersonal therapy or brief, focused analytical therapy have been shown to be effective.

Social

Decrease social isolation.

Antidepressant drugs

- Augment noradrenergic and/or serotoninergic transmission.
- Treatment duration generally six months to two years (longer if recurrent episodes).
- Established antidepressants include tricyclics and monoamine oxidase inhibitors.
- New treatments include:
  - SSRIs (Selective Serotonin Reuptake Inhibitors), e.g. citalopram, fluoxetine, paroxetine and sertraline
  - SNRIs (Serotonin/Noradrenaline Reuptake Inhibitors), e.g. venlafaxine
  - NaSSAs (Noradrenaline and Specific Serotoninergic Antidepressants), e.g. mirtazepine
  - NARIs (Noradrenaline Reuptake Inhibitors), e.g. reboxetine
  - RIMA (Reversible Inhibitors of Monoamine Oxidase-A), e.g. moclobemide.
- Advantages of newer antidepressants:
  - better tolerated
  - less cardiotoxic
  - less lethal in overdose.

Electroconvulsive therapy

Consider in severe cases unresponsive to other treatment methods.

National Service Framework suggests specialist psychiatric review in certain situations

- Unclear diagnosis.
- Complex symptoms, e.g. multiple physical problems.
- Suicide risk.
- Inadequate response to first-line treatment.
- Psychotic symptoms, e.g. delusions.

Anxiety

- Generalised anxiety disorder is characterised by frequent, persistent worry and anxiety for at least six months.
- More common in women.
- May be a new diagnosis in later life in association with other psychiatric problems such as depression, physical illness or as a side-effect of medication.
- Symptoms include:
  - poor concentration
  - irritability
  - sleep disturbance
  - fatigue
  - palpitations
  - nausea
  - shortness of breath
  - sweating
  - urinary frequency
  - headaches
  - dizziness.
- Treatment options:
  - cognitive behavioural therapy
  - relaxation therapy
  - drugs, e.g. SSRIs, short-term benzodiazepines and beta-blockers.

Sleep disturbance

Definition

Sleep disturbance is defined as any disruptive pattern of sleep such as problems falling asleep, staying asleep, excessive sleep or abnormal behaviours associated with sleep.

Statistics

- Sleep disturbance is common in older people.
- 12–25% of healthy, elderly people report chronic insomnia.
- Higher rates are seen in those with physical or psychiatric illness.
- Tends to be underdiagnosed (sufferers may incorrectly believe it is part of normal ageing) and undertreated.

Normal sleep pattern

1 NREM (non-rapid eye movement): four stages (deepest sleep in stages 3 and 4).
2 REM (rapid eye movement): dream sleep.

Factors predisposing to sleep disturbance

- Lifestyle changes, e.g. daytime inactivity with intermittent sleep episodes can lead to less fatigue at night (irregular sleeping schedule).
- Behavioural practices, e.g. association of bedtime with other activities such as reading, watching television.
- Psychiatric disorders, e.g. anxiety, depression, dementia, delirium.
- Physical illness, e.g.:
  - pain (arthritis, angina, gastro-oesophageal reflux, calf ischaemia, cramps)
  - urinary symptoms (incontinence, nocturia)
  - respiratory symptoms (congestive cardiac failure, chronic obstructive airways disease, sleep apnoea)
  - other (restless leg syndrome).
- Drugs, e.g. caffeine, alcohol, nicotine, antidepressants, antihypertensives.

Sleep history

- Identify predisposing factors.
- Establish quality, duration and timing of sleep.

Effects of sleep deprivation

- Fatigue.
- Poor concentration.
- Increased tendency to fall.
- More likely to make errors, e.g. leaving gas/electrical appliances on.

Management

Non-pharmacological

- General advice:
  - relieve contributing medical/psychiatric symptoms where possible
  - establish regular bed/awakening times
  - avoid daytime naps
  - use sleep promotion interventions, e.g. ensure quiet environment, warm drink before bed, avoid other activities while in bed.
- Cognitive behavioural therapy.
- Exercise (selected patients).

Pharmacological

- Consider low-dose sedatives in resistant cases for short periods only, e.g. 3–4 weeks.
- Sedatives are not recommended for long-term use.
- Side-effects of benzodiazepines, e.g. temazepam, include tolerance, addiction and daytime sleepiness (increases risk of falls).

Chronic schizophrenia

Definition

Chronic schizophrenia is defined as a condition characterised by disorders of thought, perception, memory and personality.

Statistics

- Majority of cases present in adolescence or early adulthood.
- Prevalence is 0.1–0.5% in over-65s.
- Cases in later life may be due to new-onset disease or life-long illness.
- 5–10% of older people have psychotic episodes – most associated with dementia; 20% due to schizophrenia.

Associations in late-onset schizophrenia

- Female gender.
- Social isolation.
- Sensory impairment (deafness/poor vision).
- Premorbid paranoid personality traits.
- *Not* associated with family history or obstetric complications as in younger onset cases.

Clinical features

- Positive symptoms:
  - delusions
  - hallucinations
  - disorganised thinking and speech.
- Negative symptoms:
  - social withdrawal
  - low motivation
  - self-neglect
  - often absent in elderly people.

Diagnosis

- Schneider's First Rank Symptoms[5] (characteristic/diagnostic features):
  - auditory hallucinations (third person, running commentary)
  - thought disorder (withdrawal, insertion, broadcasting)
  - passivity experiences (delusions of control)
  - delusional perception.
- Physical causes should be excluded.

- Differential diagnoses include:
  - dementia
  - delirium
  - depression
  - paranoid personality.

Management

Non-drug strategies

- Social interaction.
- Cognitive behavioural therapy.

Drug therapy

- Atypical antipsychotic drugs are the treatment of choice.
- Olanzepine, quetiapine and risperidone are commonly prescribed.
- These lack troublesome side-effects of typical antipsychotics such as chlorpromazine (parkinsonism, tardive dyskinesia).
- 'Start low, go slow' approach should be adopted with reference to dose and upward-titrations.
- Assistance of carers or district nurses may be required to ensure medication compliance (risperidone can be given in a long-acting intramuscular form otherwise).
- Approximately 50% of patients respond to treatment.

References

1 Department of Health (2001) *National Service Framework for Older People*. DoH, London.
2 National Institute for Clinical Excellence (2001) *Guidance on the Use of Donepezil, Rivastigmine and Galantamine for the Treatment of Alzheimer's Disease*. Technology Appraisal Guidance No. 19. Department of Health, London.
3 WHO (1992) *International Statistical Classification of Diseases and Related Health Problems*. World Health Organization, Geneva.
4 Inouye SK, van Dyck CH, Alessi CA *et al.* (1990) Clarifying confusion: the confusion assessment method. A new method for detection of delirium. *Ann Intern Med.* **113**: 941–8.
5 Schneider K (1959) *Clinical Psychopathology*. Grune and Stratton, New York.

15

Pressure sores

Definition

Pressure sores are areas of damage to skin and/or underlying tissue.

Statistics

- Ill elderly people are at high risk.
- Inpatient prevalence ranges from 5% to 10%.
- Over 70% occur in those aged over 70.
- Increase in mortality rate fivefold.
- Prolong hospital length of stay.
- Expensive to treat.
- A potential cause of litigation.
- Most can be prevented.

Common sites

- Back of head.
- Ears.
- Shoulders.
- Rib cage.
- Elbows.
- Buttocks (sacrum/ischium).
- Legs (trochanters/malleoli).
- Heels.
- Toes.

The areas affected depend on patient's position.

Grades: Agency for Health Policy and Research (1992)

Pressure sores are graded according to the degree of tissue damage.

- Grade 1
  - erythema of intact skin
  - area remains reddened for over 30 minutes after pressure is relieved.
- Grade 2
  - partial thickness skin loss involving epidermis and/or dermis.
- Grade 3
  - full thickness skin loss involving damage or necrosis to subcutaneous tissue
  - may extend to but not through fascia, bone, tendon or joint capsule.
- Grade 4
  - full thickness skin loss with damage or necrosis to muscle, bone tendon or joint capsule.

Risk factors

Intrinsic factors

- Reduced mobility, e.g. stroke/Parkinson's disease/arthritis.
- Impaired level of consciousness, e.g. neurological event/sedative medication.
- Acute illness, e.g. infection.
- Malnutrition.
- Dehydration.
- Sensory impairment, e.g. diabetes mellitus.
- Peripheral vascular disease.
- Moist skin, e.g. sweat/urine/faeces.
- Past history of pressure sores.

Extrinsic factors

- *Pressure*. Capillary occlusion compromises blood supply leading to tissue anoxia.
- *Shearing*. Superficial and deep tissue layers are forced in opposing directions, e.g. patient sliding down or being dragged up a bed or chair.

- *Friction.* Occurs when two surfaces move across each other, e.g. removal of superficial layers of skin through poor handling technique.

Prevention

- Patients should undergo a risk assessment by a trained member of staff within six hours of hospital admission.
- Pressure should be relieved with an appropriate support system.
- Skin should be inspected on a regular basis, paying particular attention to vulnerable areas.
- Frequency of repositioning should be determined by skin inspection.
- Staff should be trained in lifting techniques and the correct use of manual handling devices so that shear and friction damage can be avoided.
- Suitably trained staff, usually from the physiotherapy or occupational therapy departments, should advise regarding appropriate seating positions and aids.
- Adequate hydration and nutritional status should be maintained.
- Skin should be kept clean and dry.

Treatment

- Careful assessment of pressure sore with clear documentation of findings including site, size, grade, depth and presence of exudate/infection.
- Photograph wound if possible.
- Complete pressure relief with an appropriate device.
- Wound care (cleaning/prevention of infection/enhancement of granulation/ suitable dressings) with close liaison with tissue viability specialist nurse.
- Ensure adequate pain control.
- Optimise nutritional status (consider vitamin C and zinc).
- Minimise existing risk factors.

Pressure-relieving devices

- High-risk patients should be nursed on alternating pressure support mattresses: air-filled sacs inflate and deflate at different sites.
- Vulnerable but lower risk patients can be placed on static support systems that distribute bodyweight over a large area.
- Devices that should not be used include water-filled gloves, synthetic sheepskin and doughnut-type aids.

16

Leg ulcers

- Approximately 120 000 people in the UK have leg ulcers.
- Commonly occur in the elderly population.
- Functional capacity and quality of life can be adversely affected.
- Tissue viability services provide advice on the management of inpatients, including use of appropriate dressings, and follow patients up in an outpatient setting.
- There are three main types.

Venous ulcers

- Account for 70–80% of leg ulcers.
- Occur as a result of chronic venous insufficiency.
- Usually present on the medial surface of the lower leg.
- Surrounding skin is often pigmented.
- Bacteria often colonise ulcers – antibiotic treatment should only be employed if evidence of active infection.
- External pressure assists healing by improving venous return and reducing swelling.
- Provided there is no arterial compromise, four-layer compression bandages should be applied.
- Once healed, patients should be encouraged to wear compression stockings (assistance from a district nurse may be required for frail community-dwelling older people).
- Venous ulcers can coexist with arterial ulcers (mixed).

Arterial ulcers

- 10% of leg ulcers are due to arterial insufficiency.
- The foot and lateral aspect of the lower leg are most commonly affected.

- The leg appears pale, dusky and cold with reduced/impalpable pulses.
- Intermittent claudication is a common presenting feature, although it may not be apparent in some elderly patients as comorbidity may restrict exercise tolerance.
- Rest pain may be a feature.
- Complications include cellulitis and osteomyelitis.
- Predisposing factors are smoking, hypertension, hypercholesterolaemia and diabetes mellitus.
- Risk factor modification plays an important role in prevention/treatment.
- Ankle:brachial pressure indices <0.7 indicate an arterial component.
- Suitable patients should be referred to a vascular surgeon.

Diabetic ulcers

- Approximately 5% of ulcers are related to diabetes mellitus.
- Often occur on the foot.
- Underlying atherosclerosis and consequent vascular insufficiency are common findings.
- Cellulitis should be treated aggressively with careful observation for signs of deep-seated infection.
- Poor control of glycaemia/blood pressure/lipids, continued smoking, inadequate foot care, sensory neuropathy and badly fitting shoes are contributing factors.
- Chiropody appointments every three months are advised.

17
Hypothermia

Definition

Core body temperature <35°C.

Classification

- Mild – 35–32.2°C.
- Moderate – 32.2–28°C.
- Severe – <28°C.

Statistics

- Mortality rates for elderly people increase during winter months.
- Approximately 40 000 excess winter deaths occur in England and Wales each year.
- Majority of these are attributed to vascular (myocardial infarction/stroke) and respiratory causes.
- Cold weather induces haemoconcentration, which predisposes to thrombogenesis and impairs the body's responses to infection.
- Hypothermia is the certified cause of death in only around 300 cases per annum (and so more likely to be a secondary event).

Risk factors for hypothermia

- Medical illness (e.g. fall with long lie).
- Alcohol.
- Sedative medication.
- Poor heating.
- Inadequate finances.

Presentation

Mild

- Lethargy.
- Irritability.
- Confusion.
- Loss of fine motor co-ordination.
- Impaired judgement.
- Shivering.
- Tachycardia.
- Tachypnoea.

Moderate

- Reduced conscious level.
- Bradycardia.
- Arrhythmias (atrial fibrillation/ventricular tachycardia-fibrillation).
- Reduced respiratory rate.
- Oliguria.

Severe

- Coma.
- Arrhythmias (ventricular fibrillation/asystole).

Management

- Airway/breathing/circulation.
- Treat any precipitating underlying causes.
- Rewarming methods can include:
  - removal of wet clothing
  - blankets
  - hot air blankets
  - warm humidified oxygen
  - warm intravenous fluids.

- Prevention:
  - risk factor modification
  - education
  - care alarm
  - adequate home heating
  - financial advice and support
  - winter visits for high-risk individuals.

18

Hearing impairment/ tinnitus

Hearing impairment

Definition

- Hearing loss is the total or partial inability to hear sound in one or both ears.
- Presbyacusis (age-related hearing loss) is the progressive loss of the ability to hear high frequencies, e.g. speech.

Statistics

- Nine million people in the UK have some degree of hearing impairment.
- Hearing loss is the most common sensory impairment in the elderly.
- In 2001 in the UK:
  - 50 000 people were registered deaf
  - 144 000 were registered hard of hearing (62% aged over 75).
- Prevalence increases with age: 25% of population by 65 years, 50% by 75 years and 75% by 80 years.

Investigation

- Weber's test: a test to determine the nature of unilateral hearing loss in which a vibrating tuning fork is held against the forehead at the midline. Conduction deafness is indicated if the sound is heard more loudly in the affected ear and nerve deafness is indicated if it is heard more loudly in the normal ear.
- Rinne's test: a test to determine the ability to hear a vibrating tuning fork when it is held next to the ear and when it is placed on the mastoid process.

Diminished hearing activity through air and somewhat heightened hearing activity through bone, are suggestive of conductive deafness.

- Whisper test: a basic first-line test of hearing where the clinician whispers a number in one of the patient's ears whilst occluding the other ear, and asks the patient to repeat the number.
- Auroscopy.
- Referral for audiometry.

Classification of hearing impairment

1 Conductive deafness
 - impaired sound transmission through external canal and middle ear
 - common causes include obstruction of external auditory meatus, e.g. wax/discharge/foreign bodies, perforation of eardrum and otosclerosis.
2 Sensorineural deafness
 - secondary to cochlear or retro-cochlear pathology
 - causes include presbyacusis, Ménière's disease, drugs, e.g. gentamicin, and infection.

Management of presbyacusis

- No known cure.
- Hearing aids may help.
- Lip reading and using visual cues may aid communication.

Hearing aids

- Electronic devices consisting of a microphone, amplifier, loudspeaker and battery.
- 1.4 million people use prescribed hearing aids in England and Wales.

Communication tips

- Have the listener's attention.
- Ensure the face of the speaker is well illuminated.
- Reduce background noise.
- Maintain an optimal distance of 1 metre.
- Use a low-pitched voice.
- Speak slowly and clearly rather than shouting.
- Reword a misunderstood phrase instead of repeating.

Consequences of poor hearing

- Social isolation.
- Depression.
- Hazard risk, e.g. fire, traffic.

Tinnitus

Definition

Tinnitus is a sensation of sound arising in the head or ears. However, musical noise or words or meaningful sounds are not tinnitus and may be indicative of a psychiatric or neurological disorder.

Prevalence

- Arises with age – 14.5% are over 40 years of age and 22% are over 60 years of age.
- Majority of patients have some degree of deafness.

Aetiology

- In majority cause is unknown.
- Ménière's disease.
- Acoustic trauma.
- Chronic otitis media.
- Drug induced – aminoglycosides, chloramphenicol.
- Otosclerosis.
- Post middle-ear surgery.
- Pulsatile tinnitus – due to haemodynamic disorders.
- Involuntary contractions of palatal muscles, tympani or stapaedal muscles – the 'clicking noise' may also be heard by others.

Management

- Majority require assurance only after full assessment and investigations have been performed and a full explanation provided.

- Hearing aid for those with hearing loss may also mask tinnitus.
- Maskers.
- Electrical stimulation/suppression.
- Biofeedback.
- Support group – British Tinnitus Association.
- Antidepressants if depression present.

19

Visual impairment

Statistics

- UK figures for 2003:
  - 155 000 people registered partially sighted
  - 157 000 people registered blind.
- 30% of those aged over 65 years are estimated to be visually impaired in both eyes.
- 70% of such cases are potentially remediable.
- The incidence of visual impairment is expected to increase by 35% by 2020 as the elderly population grows.

Eye tests

- Free NHS eye examinations are available to the over-60s.
- NHS provides a domiciliary service for those who are housebound or resident in long-term care facilities.
- Advisable every two years in the elderly and annually in people with diabetes mellitus.

Registration of sight loss

- Many older people eligible for blind and partially sighted status are not registered.
- Blind registration entitles people to financial and other benefits.
- The Royal National Institute for the Blind (RNIB) can provide useful information to patients and their carers.

Consequences of poor vision

- Accidents (see driving standards).
- Falls.
- Fractures (especially hip).
- Reduced functional status and increased dependency.
- Poor quality of life.
- Social isolation.
- Depression.

Common causes of visual impairment

Refractive errors

- Can be simply corrected with glasses.
- Over 30% of visual impairment in the elderly is due solely to this.

Cataracts

- 25% of the over-75s are affected.
- The commonest treatable cause of impaired vision.
- Cataract extraction is the most common elective surgical procedure performed in older people, with 105 000 NHS operations each year.

Glaucoma

- A potential cause of blindness.
- Early detection is important.
- Prevalence in patients aged over 75 years is approximately 5%.
- Intraocular pressure can be reduced with topical miotic agents or surgery in some cases.

Age-related macular degeneration

- The most important cause of irremediable visual loss in older people.
- Over 500 000 people are affected in the UK.

- Management options include photocoagulation for the wet form and low vision aids for the dry type.

Diabetic retinopathy

- Consequences can be reduced through good glycaemic control and early detection.
- Laser treatment can be used in proliferative disease.

Department of Health Eyecare Services Steering Group (2003)

- Evidence-based care pathways for the management of low vision, cataracts, glaucoma and age-related macular degeneration have been developed
- Aims to promote a more efficient service
- Supports integration of eye care services across primary and secondary care
- Expands the role of optometrists, e.g. direct referrals to hospital eye service.

Visual standards in driving (Driver and Vehicle Licensing Agency)

- Drivers must be able to read, in good light with the aid of corrective lenses if necessary, a registration mark fixed to a motor vehicle containing letters and figures 79.4 mm high at a distance of 20.5 m (equivalent to binocular visual acuity of 6/10).
- An adequate field of vision is necessary.

20

Hypertension

Age, hypertension and cardiovascular risk

- Of Europe's population 20% are aged over 65 years.
- The 'old old' population (over 80 years) is increasing most rapidly.
- Cardiovascular disease is the single most frequent cause of death in the over-65s, is responsible for considerable morbidity and has significant cost implications for the NHS and the SSD.
- The link between hypertension and increased cardiovascular risk in the elderly is well known.
- Hypertension continues to be a significant health problem in the elderly.
- In the UK more than 50% of the 10 million people over 65 years old are hypertensive.
- Elderly hypertensive patients are now seen as an important target group who appear to benefit from antihypertensive treatment in terms of improved outcomes.
- Intervention trials have demonstrated that antihypertensive treatment in older patients can reduce the incidence of stroke by 30%, coronary heart disease by 20% and all vascular deaths by nearly 25%.
- An aggressive approach to blood pressure lowering is warranted up to at least the age of 80, particularly in those at increased cardiovascular risk.
- The absolute benefit from treatment in the elderly is much larger than that for younger patients with hypertension because of their higher absolute risk.

Isolated systolic hypertension (ISH)

- A distinct pathological entity resulting in systolic blood pressures (SBP) > 160 mmHg and diastolic blood pressures (DBP) < 90 mmHg.
- Prevalence increases with age (8% in the over-60s and 25% in those over 80 years).

- The Framingham Heart Study showed that among hypertensive people aged over 65, 70% had ISH rather than combined systolic and diastolic hypertension.
- A better predictor of cardiovascular events than DBP.

British Hypertension Society guidelines (2004)[1]

- Routine investigations should include:
  - urinalysis
  - serum electrolyes and creatinine
  - plasma glucose
  - serum total:HDL cholesterol
  - 12-lead ECG.
- Use non-pharmacological measures in all hypertensive and borderline hypertensive people with sustained SBP over 160 mmHg or sustained DBP over 100 mmHg.
- Initiate antihypertensive drug therapy in people with sustained SBP over 160 mmHg or sustained DBP over 100 mmHg.
- Decide on treatment in people with sustained SBP between 140 and 159 mmHg or sustained DBP between 90 and 99 mmHg according to the presence and/or absence of target organ damage, cardiovascular disease or a 10-year coronary heart disease risk of more than 20%.
- In non-diabetic hypertensive people, optimal BP targets are SBP < 140 mmHg and DBP < 85 mmHg.
- In diabetic hypertensive people, optimal BP targets are SBP < 140 mmHg and DBP < 80 mmHg.
- In the absence of contraindications or compelling indications for other antihypertensive agents, low-dose thiazide diuretics or beta-blockers are preferred as first-line therapy for the majority of hypertensive people.
- In the absence of compelling indications for beta-blockade, diuretics or long-acting dihydropyridine calcium antagonists are preferred to beta-blockers in older subjects.
- Combination therapy will be required to achieve recommended BP targets in many cases.
- Other drugs that reduce cardiovascular risk should be considered (aspirin for secondary prevention of cardiovascular disease and primary prevention in treated hypertensive patients over 50 years who have a 10-year risk > 15% and statins for hypertensive people with cardiovascular disease

irrespective of cholesterol level and for primary prevention in those with a 10-year risk of $\geq 20\%$.

- Evidence for benefit from antihypertensive treatment extends until at least the age of 80, and regular BP screening should continue until this age.
- Once started, antihypertensive treatment should be continued after patients reach the age of 80.
- When hypertension is first diagnosed beyond the age of 80, there is no firm evidence to guide policy, but decisions should probably be based on biological rather than chronological age.
- Patients with newly diagnosed hypertension after the age of 80 should be considered for treatment, provided they are generally fit and have a reasonable life expectancy, particularly if they have hypertensive complications.
- Elderly hypertensives respond to non-pharmacological measures to lower BP at least as well as young patients.
- Antihypertensive treatment is indicated and clearly beneficial in people over 60 years when BP averages are > 160 mmHg systolic and > 90 mmHg diastolic.

Treatment

- Hypertension is worth treating at least up to the age of 80 with benefits not only for cardiovascular death but also possibly for cognitive decline and dementia.
- Elderly hypertensives represent a special group with particular needs and antihypertensive prescribing in this group represents both a clinical and practical challenge.

Non-pharmacological treatment

- Lifestyle modification:
  - weight loss
  - regular exercise
  - reduced use of salt
  - increased intake of fruit and vegetables
  - limited alcohol consumption.

Drug therapy

- Agents should be appropriate to the patient's comorbidities.
- World Health Organization (WHO)/International Society of Hypertension (ISH) guidelines recognise all classes of antihypertensive agent as suitable first-line therapy, but they and the BHS guidelines recommend long-acting calcium channel antagonists in older patients, particularly for the treatment of ISH.
- Although thiazide diuretics are commonly prescribed and are of proven benefit in some patients, there are certain drawbacks (low tolerability, low efficacy in reversing LVH and lack of glucose and lipid neutrality).
- The ideal agent for the elderly hypertensive patient would:
  - be supported by accepted guidelines
  - be effective against concomitant risk factors
  - offer simple once-daily dosing
  - have good tolerability
  - be unlikely to prompt non-compliance
  - be cost-effective.

British Hypertension Society 'AB/CD' treatment recommendations

- Young and Caucasian patients usually have renin-dependent hypertension that responds to treatment with ACE-Inhibitors or Angiotensin II Receptor Antagonists (A) or B-blockers (B).
- Older or non-Caucasian patients who may not have renin-dependent hypertension should be treated with calcium channel blockers (C) or diuretics (D).
- If a second agent is required, (A) or (B) should be combined with (C) or (D).
- If a third agent is necessary, (A), (C) and (D) should be used in combination.
- Combined use of (B) and (D) should be avoided because of increased insulin resistance.

Management problems in the elderly hypertensive patient

- Elderly hypertensive patients can present a considerable management challenge.

- Salt restriction is difficult to practise in view of diminished taste sensation.
- Compliance with weight loss and diet restrictions is often unsuccessful.
- Coexisting diseases preclude certain drug choices.
- Disturbance in cognitive function may affect drug compliance.
- Polypharmacy can lead to drug interactions, drug-related side-effects and medication non-compliance.

Key trials

Treatment of hypertension in the elderly has been shown in several randomised controlled trials to significantly reduce cardiovascular mortality. In the very elderly (over 80 years), due to the limited amount of experimental data, the benefit of treating this age group is not clearly demonstrated. However, trials targeting this age group are under way and should provide evidence as to whether it is worth treating the very elderly hypertensive.

- SHEP: SHEP Co-operative Research Group (1991) Prevention of stroke by antihypertensive drug treatment in older persons with isolated systolic hypertension. Final results of the Systolic Hypertension in the Elderly Program (SHEP). *JAMA*. **265**: 3255–64.
- SYST-EUR: Staessen JA, Fagard R, Thijs L *et al*. (1997) Randomised double-blind comparison of placebo and active treatment for older patients with isolated systolic hypertension. The Systolic Hypertension in Europe (Syst-Eur) Trial Investigators. *Lancet*. **350**: 757–64.
- HOT: Hansson L, Zanchetti A, Carruthers SG *et al*. for the HOT Study Group (1998) Effects of intensive blood-pressure lowering and low-dose aspirin in patients with hypertension: principal results of the Hypertension Optimal Treatment (HOT) randomised trial. *Lancet*. **351**: 1755–62.
- SYST-CHINA: Liu L, Wang JG, Gong L, Liu G, Staessen JA (1998) Comparison of active treatment and placebo in older Chinese patients with isolated systolic hypertension. Systolic Hypertension in China (Syst-China) Collaborative Group. *J Hypertens*. **16**: 1823–9.
- CAPPP: Hansson L, Lindholm LH, Niskanen L *et al*. (1999a) Effect of angiotensin-converting enzyme inhibition compared with conventional therapy on cardiovascular morbidity and mortality in hypertension: the Captopril Prevention Project (CAPPP) randomised trial. *Lancet*. **353**: 611–14.
- STOP-2: Hansson L, Lindholm LH, Ekbom T *et al*. (1999b) Randomised trial of old and new antihypertensive drugs in elderly patients: cardiovascular mortality and morbidity in the Swedish Trial in Old Patients with Hypertension-2 Study. *Lancet*. **354**: 1751–6.

- HOPE: Yusuf S, Sleight P, Pogue J *et al.* (2000) Effects of an angiotensin-converting enzyme inhibitor, ramipril, on cardiovascular events in high-risk patients. The Heart Outcomes Prevention Evaluation Study (HOPE). *N Engl J Med.* **342**: 145–53.
- UKPDS: United Kingdom Prospective Diabetes Study Group (1999) Tight blood pressure control and risk of macrovascular and microvascular complications in Type 2 diabetes (UKPDS 38). *Br Med J.* **318**: 29.
- INSIGHT: Brown NJ, Palmer CR, Castaigne A *et al.* (2000) Morbidity and mortality in patients randomised to double-blind treatment with a long-acting calcium channel blocker or diuretic in the International Nifedipine GITS Study: Intervention as a Goal in Hypertension Treatment (INSIGHT). *Lancet.* **356**: 366–72.
- NORDIL: Hansson L, Hedner T, Lund-Johansen P *et al.* (2000a) Randomised effects of calcium antagonists compared with diuretics and beta-blockers on cardiovascular morbidity and mortality in hypertension: the Nordic Diltiazem (NORDIL) Study. *Lancet.* **356**: 359–65.

Reference

1 Guidelines for the management of hypertension: a report of the fourth working party of the British Hypertension Society (2004) *Journal of Human Hypertension.* **18**: 139–85.

21

Heart failure

Definition (NICE 2003)[1]

Heart failure is a complex syndrome that can result from any structural or functional disorder that impairs the ability of the heart to function as a pump to support a physiological circulation.

Classification (New York Heart Association)[2]

I   No symptoms on ordinary activity.
II Slight limitation of physical activity (comfortable at rest but ordinary activity results in fatigue and shortness of breath).
III Marked limitation of physical activity (comfortable at rest but less than ordinary activity causes symptoms).
IV Dyspnoeic at rest.

Statistics

- 1–2% of UK population have heart failure.
- Median age of presentation is 76 years.
- Prevalence increases with advancing age – less than 1% of people under 65 years are affected compared to 10–20% of the over-80s.
- More common in men than women (2:1).
- Accounts for 5% of all medical admissions.
- Readmission rates over a three-month period are around 50%.
- Number of cases is projected to rise with time.
- Prognosis is poor with an annual mortality rate of 10–50% depending on severity.

National Service Framework for Coronary Heart Disease: Chapter Six – Heart Failure (2000)[3]

Aims

- To help patients with heart failure live longer and achieve better quality of life.
- To help patients with unresponsive heart failure receive appropriate palliative care support.

Standard

- Doctors should arrange for people with suspected heart failure to be offered appropriate investigations that will confirm or refute the diagnosis.
- For those in whom heart failure is confirmed, its cause should be identified and the treatments most likely to both relieve symptoms and reduce risk of death should be offered.

Common causes

- Ischaemic heart disease.
- Hypertension.
- Valvular heart disease.
- Arrhythmias.
- Cardiomyopathies.
- Alcohol.

Elderly patients can suffer acute cardiac decompensation following a non-cardiac illness, e.g. pneumonia.

Diagnosis

European Society of Cardiology diagnostic criteria for chronic heart failure (2001)[4]

1 Symptoms of heart failure at rest or during exercise (dyspnoea, reduced exercise tolerance, orthopnoea, peripheral oedema).
2 Objective evidence of cardiac dysfunction.
3 Response to appropriate treatment.

- Elderly patients may not present with classic symptoms and signs, making the diagnosis challenging.
- Typical features, including leg swelling and shortness of breath, have a wide differential diagnosis including:

Peripheral oedema
Venous insufficiency
Drug-induced fluid retention
Hypoalbuminaemia
Inactivity
Lymphoedema

Dyspnoea
Chronic obstructive airways disease
Pulmonary embolus
Anaemia

BNP

- B-type natriuretic peptide.
- Serum level is raised in patients with heart failure.
- Negative predictive value of 98% makes heart failure a very unlikely diagnosis if level is low.

Other baseline tests

- Renal/thyroid/liver function.
- Full blood count.
- Fasting glucose and lipid profile.
- Urinalysis.
- Chest x-ray.
- ECG.
- Echocardiogram.

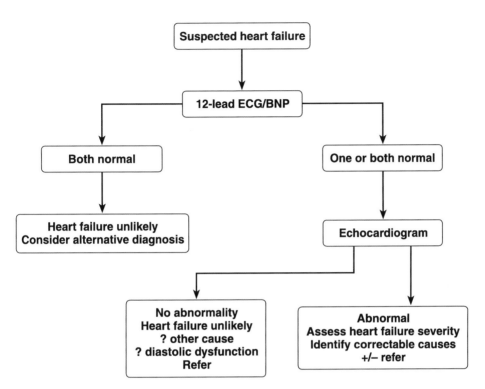

Figure 21.1   From NICE guidelines for diagnosis of heart failure.[1]

Management

Non-pharmacological

- Fluid and dietary salt restriction to maintain a stable weight.
- Regular gentle exercise as tolerated.
- Cessation of smoking.
- Limited alcohol.
- Optimisation of blood pressure control.
- Annual influenza vaccination.

Pharmacological

Medication concordance is essential.

Diuretics

- Improve symptoms.
- No survival benefit when used alone.
- Doses can be adjusted according to requirements.
- Most patients will need a loop diuretic at some stage.
- A thiazide can be used in combination with a loop for powerful synergistic effect.
- For spironolactone see below.

Angiotensin converting enzyme inhibitors (ACE-I)

- Improve symptoms.
- Reduce mortality rate.
- Should be considered in all cases of left ventricular systolic impairment (ejection fraction <40%).
- Contraindications include severe aortic stenosis, bilateral renal artery stenosis and significant renal dysfunction.
- Monitor renal function (U+E before first dose, 1–2 weeks after each dose increment, then 3–6 monthly).
- Aim to use recommended target doses, e.g. ramipril 5 mg bd; perindopril 4 mg od.

Angiotensin II receptor antagonists

- Consider if ACE-I not tolerated.

Beta-blockers

- Improve survival.
- Consider once stable on diuretic and ACE-1.
- Bisoprolol and carvedilol are licensed for use in heart failure in the UK.
- Start at a low dose and increase slowly as tolerated over weeks/months.

Spironolactone

- An aldosterone antagonist potassium-sparing diuretic.
- Reduces mortality rate in patients with moderate/severe heart failure (New York Heart Association Classes III/IV) when combined with a conventional diuretic and ACE-I.

Digoxin

- For ventricular rate control in atrial fibrillation.
- Exerts a positive inotropic effect and so can be used for patients in sinus rhythm with severe left ventricular failure.
- Does not reduce mortality rate.

Vasodilators

- A nitrate/hydralazine combination can be used if intolerant of ACE-I/angiotensin II receptor antagonists.

Inotropes

- Can be considered for acutely unwell inpatients unresponsive to conventional therapy.

Other interventions in selected patients

- Coronary revascularisation.
- Cardiac resynchronisation (biventricular pacing).
- Implantable cardioverter defibrillators.

Follow-up

- Cardiology, general medical or geriatric clinics.
- Nurse-led heart failure monitoring service.
- Assessment should include:
    - symptom review
    - examination
    - weight
    - medication optimisation
    - compliance assurance
    - dietary/fluid modifications
    - renal function
    - education of patient and carer.

Prognosis

- Worse than for some forms of cancer.
- Should be discussed with patients and their carers.
- Need to focus not just on treatments that prolong life, but on those that relieve symptoms and improve quality of life.
- Skills of palliative care professionals should be translated into caring for patients with severe heart failure.

Diastolic heart failure

- Patients with symptoms of heart failure but normal left ventricular function on echocardiography.
- Affects 1% of elderly population.
- Little evidence on best treatment approach.
- Aim to control blood pressure, relieve symptoms of fluid overload and prevent ischaemia.

References

1 National Institute for Clinical Excellence (2003) *Chronic Heart Failure in Adults in Primary and Secondary Care. A clinical guideline for the NHS in England and Wales.* NICE, London.
2 The Criteria Committee of the New York Heart Association (1994) *Nomenclature and Criteria for Diagnosis of Diseases of the Heart and Blood Vessels* (9e). Little, Brown and Company, Boston, MA, 253–6.
3 Department of Health (2000) *National Service Framework for Coronary Heart Disease.* DoH, London.
4 European Society of Cardiology (2001) The taskforce for the diagnosis and treatment of chronic heart failure. *Eur Heart J.* **22**: 1527–60.

22

Atrial fibrillation

Definition

- Unco-ordinated electrical activity of the atria resulting in little/no effective mechanical contraction.
- Manifested on ECG as absence of P waves and irregular baseline of fibrillatory waves.

Pathophysiology

- Initiated by rapid electrical discharges from atrial cells.
- Various trigger sites including cuffs of muscle at openings of pulmonary veins, atrial appendages and coronary sinus.
- Structural changes develop in atria over time (enlargement, fibrosis and hypertrophy) which perpetuate arrhythmogenesis.

Classification

- *Persistent*: does not terminate spontaneously/present for <1 year.
- *Paroxysmal*: terminates spontaneously but recurs.
- *Permanent*: cannot be terminated by either chemical or electrical cardioversion/persists for >1 year.

Statistics

- Commonest cardiac arrhythmia.
- Affects 0.4% total population.

- Prevalence increases with age:
  - <1% <60 years
  - 6–10% >80 years.
- Substantial risk of thromboembolic stroke:
  - risk of ischaemic stroke increased 2–7-fold in non-rheumatic cases
  - risk increases 17-fold in rheumatic atrial fibrillation (AF).

Common causes

- Lone AF (no identifiable cause).
- Valvular heart disease, especially mitral valve.
- Hypertension.
- Ischaemic heart disease.
- Hyperthyroidism.
- Alcohol.

Clinical features

- Patients may be asymptomatic.
- Symptoms include palpitations, shortness of breath, fatigue, chest pain, dizziness and syncope.
- Cardiac ischaemia, heart failure and thromboembolic events may be precipitated.

Management

- Where possible the underlying cause should be corrected.
- Two important aspects to treatment:
  - rate control ± restoration of sinus rhythm
  - prevention of thromboembolism.

Rate control

- Digoxin, rate-limiting calcium channel antagonists, beta-blockers and amiodarone are agents commonly used to control ventricular rate by slowing conduction through the atrioventricular node.
- Little evidence that restoration of sinus rhythm is more favourable than rate control and anticoagulation but it may help relieve symptoms.

- Sinus rhythm can be regained pharmacologically (e.g. amiodarone, flecainide, propafenone) or electrically.
- Direct current (DC) electrical shock requires anticoagulation with International Normalised Ratio (INR) maintained at 2–3 for at least three weeks when AF has been present for >48 hours (unless transoesophageal echocardiography excludes thrombus).
- Long-term maintenance of sinus rhythm after DC cardioversion is poor (approximately 1/5 over five years).
- DC cardioversion success rates may be enhanced by drug prophylaxis, e.g. amiodarone, flecainide.

Prevention of thromboembolism

- One in six patients who has a stroke is in AF.
- Additional risk factors include:
  - age >75
  - previous stroke
  - transient ischaemic attacks (TIAs)
  - structural heart disease
  - hypertension
  - ischaemic heart disease with left ventricular dysfunction
  - diabetes mellitus.
- Risk of ischaemic stroke can be reduced with antiplatelet agents or anticoagulation.
- Aspirin at a dose of 300mg/day decreases risk by 20%.
- Warfarin (optimum INR 2–3) reduces risk by 60–70%.
- As warfarin carries a small risk of bleeding, a risk versus benefit decision needs to be made in each case.
- Tight control INR reduces bleeding tendency.
- High-risk patients should be offered warfarin therapy assuming no contraindications preclude its use.
- Cautions/contraindications to warfarin include:
  - recent trauma/surgery/haemorrhage
  - actively bleeding gastrointestinal lesion
  - uncontrolled hypertension
  - falls
  - alcohol misuse
  - severe renal/hepatic impairment
  - moderate/severe cognitive impairment
  - likely non-compliance
  - warfarin allergy (consider nicoumalone as an alternative).

- Therapy guideline:

  1. <60 years   –   aspirin 300 mg/day
     no risk factors
  2. 60–74 years   –   aspirin 300 mg/day
     no risk factors
  3. >75 years   –   warfarin (INR 2–3 or 3–4
     risk factors   for prosthetic heart valves)
     no warfarin contraindications

- Elderly people are often inappropriately denied warfarin therapy on grounds of age alone.
- Decisions regarding continued warfarin use in older people should be reviewed as clinical situations may change over time, e.g. new falls.
- INR can be monitored in hospital anticoagulation clinics, GP surgeries or at home with the aid of district nurse services.

23
Stroke

Definition (WHO 1980)

A clinical syndrome typified by rapidly developing signs of focal (at times global) disturbance of cerebral function, lasting more than 24 hours or leading to death within 24 hours, with no apparent cause other than that of vascular origin.

Statistics

- Third commonest cause of death and most frequent cause of severe disability worldwide.
- Incidence increases with age and is expected to rise by 20% over the next 20 years as population ages.
- Accounts for 12% of deaths in the UK.
- 110 000 people (2 per 1000) have a first stroke in England and Wales each year.
- Past history of stroke or transient ischaemic attack (TIA) increases the risk of further event 13–15-fold.
- 30% of patients die during the first month.
- 35% are significantly disabled at one year.
- 5% are admitted to long-term care.
- Mortality and morbidity rates are higher in the elderly population.
- Stroke care costs the NHS over £2 billion per year.

Classification

- 85% ischaemic:
  - atherosclerotic 20%
  - penetrating artery disease 25%
  - cardiogenic embolism 20%

- cryptogenic 30%
- others (e.g. prothrombotic states, carotid artery dissection) 5%.
- Clinical syndromes depend on affected vascular territory:
  - total anterior circulation infarction (TACI) – territory supplied by middle cerebral artery (MCA)
  - partial anterior circulation infarction (PACI) – occlusion of branches of MCA or isolated anterior cerebral artery occlusion
  - posterior circulation infarction (POCI) – infarction of brainstem, cerebellum or occipital lobe
  - lacunar infarct (LACI) – occlusion of basal perforating arteries.
- 15% haemorrhagic:
  - intraparenchymal
  - subarachnoid.

Risk factors

- Age.
- Male gender.
- Afro–Caribbean and South Asian ethnic groups.
- Low socioeconomic class.
- Previous stroke.
- History of TIA.
- Atrial fibrillation.
- Carotid artery stenosis.
- Valvular heart disease.
- Hypertension.
- Hypercholesterolaemia.
- Smoking.
- Diabetes mellitus.
- Alcohol misuse.
- Physical inactivity.

Consequences of stroke

- Aspiration.
- Cognitive impairment.
- Communication difficulties.
- Contractures.
- Deep venous thrombosis/pulmonary embolus.
- Dependency.

- Depression.
- Disability.
- Dysphagia.
- Incontinence (urinary/faecal).
- Infection (chest/urine).
- Pain (mechanical/neuropathic).
- Pressure sores.

Primary prevention

- Control of blood pressure.
- Antiplatelet/anticoagulant therapy for atrial fibrillation.
- Carotid endarterectomy in suitable patients.
- Smoking cessation.
- Moderate alcohol consumption.
- Low fat/salt intake.
- Exercise.

Acute management

Antiplatelet therapy

- Aspirin is recommended as soon as possible after onset of symptoms (can be given rectally or via nasogastric tube if necessary).
- Can be administered to patients with suspected ischaemic stroke even when CT brain confirmation is not available (CT should be performed within 48 hours of admission).
- Evidence for doses of 50–300 mg daily.
- Prompt treatment reduces risk of further stroke or death in hospital and risk of death and dependency at six months.

Thrombolysis

- Alteplase is licensed for use in UK.
- Haemorrhage must be excluded by CT or MRI brain before administration.
- Improves outcome if administered to selected patients within three hours of acute ischaemic stroke onset by an experienced stroke physician in a specialist centre.

- Patients 30% more likely to have minimal/no disability three months post-stroke.
- Significantly reduces length of hospital stay.
- Main complication is intracranial haemorrhage.
- Contraindications:
  - active internal bleeding
  - intracranial or intraspinal surgery, serious head injury or stroke within previous three months
  - intracranial neoplasm, arteriovenous malformation or aneurysm
  - severe uncontrolled hypertension
  - bleeding diathesis
  - warfarin with INR more than 1.7
  - heparin therapy with elevated Activated Partial Thromboplastin Time (APTT)
  - platelet count less than 100.
- Widespread use is limited until results of ongoing trials published and adequate resources allocated.

Early management

Nutrition

- Malnutrition is associated with worse outcome.
- Patients with an unsafe swallow should have a nasogastric tube inserted for feeding.

Bowel and bladder

- Double incontinence is common in severe strokes.
- See Chapter 25 on bowel and bladder management.

Positioning

- Important in prevention of pressure sores, contractures and pneumonia.

Deep vein thrombosis prophylaxis

- Ensure adequate hydration.
- Immobile patients should wear compression stockings if no contra-indications.
- Subcutaneous heparin increases risk of intracerebral haemorrhage and so should not be used routinely.

Rehabilitation

Stroke units

Designated stroke units offering a multidisciplinary approach to stroke care and led by a physician with a specialist interest in stroke have been shown to reduce mortality, dependency and need for institutionalisation without prolonging length of stay.

Multidisciplinary team

- Physician specialising in stroke medicine.
- Clinical nurse specialist.
- Stroke care co-ordinator.
- Speech and language therapist.
- Physiotherapist.
- Occupational therapist.
- Dietician.
- Clinical psychologist.
- Continence advisor.
- Pharmacist.
- Social worker.
- Translators.

Secondary prevention (National Clinical Guidelines 2004)[1]

- Risk of further stroke is approximately 7% per year.
- Patients are at highest risk in early stages.

Control of hypertension

- Minimum accepted blood pressure (BP) is 150/90.
- British Hypertension Society guidelines suggest optimal BP of < 140/85 (130/80 in patients with diabetes mellitus).
- Treatment should be commenced if BP remains elevated after two weeks.
- Combination of a long-acting ACE inhibitor, e.g. ramipril or perindopril and thiazide diuretic, e.g. indapamide, should be considered as first line.

Prevention of thromboembolism

- Patients with ischaemic stroke who are not anticoagulated should be taking antiplatelet therapy, e.g. aspirin 50–300 mg od, clopidogrel 75 mg od or a combination of low-dose aspirin and modified-release dipyridamole (200 mg bd).
- Patients who have had an event while taking aspirin alone and in whom anticoagulation is not appropriate should be prescribed clopidogrel in addition or switched to dipyridamole modified release.
- After 14 days, warfarin should be prescribed for patients in atrial fibrillation assuming haemorrhage has been excluded and no contraindications exist.
- Patients with carotid artery area stroke, carotid artery stenosis greater than 70% and minor/no residual disability should be considered for carotid endarterectomy, angioplasty or stent insertion.

Anti-lipid treatment

- Consider statin therapy if total cholesterol > 3.5 mmol/l.

Lifestyle advice

- Smoking cessation.
- Avoiding excess alcohol.
- Low-fat diet.
- Reducing salt intake.
- Exercise.

Discharge planning

- Close liaison between disciplines.
- Communication of information to GP and community services.

Long-term management

- Outpatient follow-up (further input may be required after active rehabilitation phase).
- Ensure maintenance of risk factor modification.
- Monitor for development of complications.
- Support for informal carers.

Carers

Informal carers need:

- information and education about all aspects of stroke
- to be involved in decision making
- emotional, financial, practical and social support
- a named contact for advice/assistance in crises
- details of support groups, e.g. Stroke Association
- opportunities for respite.

National Service Framework for Older People: Standard 5: Stroke (2001)[2]

Aims

- To reduce incidence of stroke.
- To ensure stroke sufferers have prompt access to integrated stroke care services.

Milestones for 2004

- GPs should identify and treat patients at risk of stroke.
- GPs should use a protocol agreed with local specialists for rapid referral for management of TIAs.

- GPs should identify those who have had a stroke and treat according to locally agreed protocols.
- GPs should have established clinical audit systems for stroke.
- All general hospitals caring for patients with stroke should have a specialised stroke service.

Transient ischaemic attack

- A thromboembolic event resulting in sudden onset of focal cerebral or retinal deficit that recovers within 24 hours.
- Duration usually less than 30 minutes.
- Source of thromboembolism most commonly carotid artery, heart, aorta or vertebrobasilar vessels.
- A warning sign for future stroke (15% of ischaemic strokes preceded by TIA).
- Risk of stroke following TIA:
  - 8–12% at seven days
  - 11–15% at one month
  - 17–18% at three months.
- Formal assessment, modification of risk factors and initiation of preventive therapy should occur at earliest opportunity.
- CT brain is not necessary before prescribing prophylaxis.
- Aspirin recommended as first line for patients in sinus rhythm (clopidogrel if aspirin intolerant).
- For patients in sinus rhythm already taking aspirin, addition of a second recommended antiplatelet agent is suggested if recurrent TIAs.
- Warfarin is more effective than aspirin in prevention of stroke in people with atrial fibrillation (not recommended for patients in sinus rhythm).

References

1 Department of Health (2001) *National Service Framework for Older People*. DoH, London.
2 Royal College of Physicians (2004) *National Clinical Guidelines for Stroke*. RCP, London.

24

Parkinson's disease

Statistics

- One of the commonest neurological conditions affecting older people.
- 160/100 000 population are affected.
- Prevalence increases with age (2% of over-80s).
- Annual incidence 13/100 000.

Pathology

- Degeneration of dopaminergic neurones in substantia nigra.
- Precise aetiology unknown.
- Causes of parkinsonism but not true Parkinson's disease include cerebrovascular disease and drugs, e.g. neuroleptics.

Clinical features

Parkinson's disease has four cardinal signs:

1 tremor
2 rigidity
3 bradykinesia
4 loss of postural reflexes.

Diagnosis

United Kingdom Parkinson's Disease Society diagnostic criteria

- Diagnosis of parkinsonism requires bradykinesia plus at least one of:
  - muscular rigidity
  - rest tremor
  - postural instability.
- Exclusion criteria:
  - recurrent strokes
  - repeated head injuries
  - encephalitis.
- Supportive criteria:
  - unilateral onset
  - evidence of progression
  - persistent asymmetry
  - excellent response to L-dopa
  - severe L-dopa induced chorea
  - L-dopa response for more than five years
  - clinical course more than 10 years.
- Accurate diagnosis may be complicated by comorbidity, e.g. cerebro-vascular disease, osteoarthritis or atypical presentation.
- Specialist referral advised.

Consequences

Physical

- Falls.
- Postural hypotension.
- Pressure sores.
- Urinary incontinence.
- Constipation.
- Dysphagia.
- Aspiration pneumonia.
- Dysarthria.

Psychiatric

- Depression.
- Cognitive impairment.

Social

- Loss of independence.
- Isolation.

Management

Drug therapy

- L-dopa commonly prescribed as a first-line agent in combination with a dopa-decarboxylase inhibitor (risk of developing motor complications over time).
- Dopaminergic agonists, e.g. ropinerole, pramipexole, pergolide can be used as monotherapy or as adjuncts to L-dopa (less likely to cause dyskinetic side-effects).
- Other therapeutic agents include monoamine oxidase-type B inhibitors, e.g. selegiline, and catechol-o-methyltransferase inhibitors, e.g. entacapone.

Multidisciplinary team

Care should be provided by a geriatrician with a special interest in Parkinson's disease or a neurologist in close liaison with other professionals:

- specialist nurse
- physiotherapist
- occupational therapist
- speech and language therapist
- psychologist +/− psychiatrist
- pharmacist
- social worker.

Parkinson's disease nurse specialists

- Offer information and support for patients and their carers.
- Monitor effects of medication.
- Anticipate potential problems.
- Provide continuity of care and a link between primary and secondary care services.

25

Bowel and bladder management

Bowel

Constipation

Definition

Constipation is defined as self-reporting of two or more of the following symptoms on more than 25% of occasions in the prior three months:

- two or fewer bowel movements per week
- hard stools
- straining
- feeling of incomplete evacuation.

Prevalence

- Self-reported constipation increases with age, and older people with constipation primarily tend to have difficulty with rectal evacuation, straining and hard stools.
- Very common in immobilised older persons in whom gastrocolic reflex (peristalsis resulting from food entering the stomach) is impaired.

Causes

- Low dietary fibre.
- Dehydration.
- Immobility.
- Drugs, e.g. opiates, calcium channel blockers, diuretics, anticholinergic agents.

- Colorectal disease, e.g. diverticular disease, neoplasm.
- Metabolic conditions, e.g. hypothyroidism, diabetes mellitus, hypercalcaemia.
- Neurological pathology, e.g. stroke, Parkinson's disease, spinal cord injury.
- Depression.

Management

- Consider above causes and investigate where appropriate.
- In cases of chronic constipation:
  - increase fibre intake
  - increase fluid intake if possible
  - increase physical activity if able
  - stop constipating medications if feasible
  - people with limited mobility or those living in a residential/nursing home: stimulant laxative such as senna or stool softener such as Docusate, on an intermittent basis
  - those with impaction may require suppositories (glycerine or bisacodyl) or enemas (microlax then phosphate)
  - if enemas are unsuccessful, proceed to manual evacuation or rectal washouts.

Diarrhoea

Definition

Diarrhoea is the passage of more than 300 ml liquid faeces in 24 hours.

Causes

- Constipation with overflow.
- Drugs, e.g. laxatives, antibiotics.
- Infection, e.g. viral, bacterial, parasitic.
- Gastrointestinal pathology, e.g. inflammatory bowel disease, malabsorption.

Management

- Exclude faecal impaction.
- Stop contributing medications if possible.
- Send stool specimen for analysis if appropriate (MCS, *Clostridium difficile*, OCP).

- Investigate for gastrointestinal cause if clinically indicated.
- Rehydrate as necessary.
- Antidiarrhoeal agents may be required, e.g. codeine phosphate, loperamide.

Faecal incontinence

Definition

Faecal incontinence is the involuntary leakage of rectal contents through the anal canal.

Statistics

- Affects 2% of adult population.
- Higher prevalence in elderly population:
  - community dwellers up to 6%
  - residents of residential/nursing homes up to 30%.
- Underdetected and so undertreated.

Contributing factors

- Loose stool.
- Faecal impaction with overflow.
- Medication.
- Poor mobility (inability to reach toilet in time).
- Damage to anal sphincter/pelvic floor (e.g. obstetric causes especially forceps delivery, surgical procedures).
- Comorbidities, e.g. stroke, dementia.

Consequences

- Skin irritation/infection.
- Social isolation.
- Depression.
- Anxiety.
- Carer stress.
- Institutionalisation.

Management

- Increase awareness among health professionals.
- Investigate and treat contributing causes.

- Regular toileting.
- Adequately positioned toilet facilities.

Bladder

Urinary incontinence

Definition

An involuntary loss of urine at least twice per week irrespective of amount lost.

Statistics

- More common with ageing but not a normal feature of ageing.
- Prevalence:
  - 10–35% of community dwellers aged over 65 years
  - 25–30% of elderly inpatients and those in residential care
  - 50% of nursing home residents
  - 70% of patients in continuing care.
- Many symptoms are unreported.

Age-related changes in lower urinary tract

- Decrease in:
  - bladder capacity
  - ability to postpone voiding
  - urinary flow rate
  - urethral closing pressure.
- Increase in:
  - post-void residual volume
  - prostate size
  - involuntary detrusor contractions
  - nocturnal urine excretion.

Consequences

- Social isolation.
- Depression.
- Anxiety.
- Carer stress.

- Financial burden.
- Rashes.
- Skin infections.
- Precipitating factor for institutionalisation.

Associated conditions

- Arthritis.
- Stroke.
- Parkinson's disease.
- Cognitive impairment.
- Peripheral vascular disease.
- Venous insufficiency.
- Constipation.
- Congestive cardiac failure.
- Chronic lung disease.
- Diabetes mellitus.

Classification

Acute

- Acronym (DIAPPERS):
  - D Delirium
  - I Infection/intercurrent illness
  - A Atrophic urethritis/vaginitis
  - P Pharmacological/drugs
  - P Psychological
  - E Excessive urine, e.g. fluid intake, diuretics, diabetes mellitus, hypercalcaemia
  - R Restricted mobility
  - S Stool impaction.

Chronic

1 Detrusor instability
   - Commonest cause of urinary incontinence in older people regardless of gender.
   - Affects 10–30% of older women.
   - Involuntary uninhibited detrusor contractions overcome sphincter mechanisms.
   - May be idiopathic, obstructive or neuropathic.

- Exacerbated by anxiety or fast bladder filling, e.g. after diuretics.
- Symptoms include urgency, urge incontinence, night-time incontinence, frequency (patients void repeatedly to avoid incontinence – more than 7 times/24 hours) and nocturia.
- Treatment options include:
  (i) behavioural modification:
    - aim to decrease urinary frequency to acceptable level and increase bladder volume
    - modify diet and fluid intake (avoid caffeine, four pints of fluid per day – fluid restriction increases bladder instability and risk of urinary tract infection)
    - ensure regular bowel habit
    - bladder retraining:
      (a) aim to suppress urge to void
      (b) time between voiding is lengthened leading to increased bladder capacity and fewer incontinent episodes
      (c) continue until voiding interval is 3–4 hours
      (d) usually takes weeks or months
      (e) requires patient motivation and intact cognitive function
      (f) prompted/scheduled voiding can be used in demented patients.
  (ii) drugs:
    - mainstay of treatment
    - contraction of detrusor mediated by stimulation of muscarinic receptors in bladder wall by acetylcholine
    - oxybutynin has anticholinergic and direct smooth muscle relaxant properties that reduce intravesical pressure, increase bladder capacity and decrease frequency of contraction
    - side-effects (dry mouth, blurred vision, nausea, constipation) may lead to dose reduction or withdrawal
    - slow-release formulation (oxybutynin-XL) is often better tolerated
    - tolterodine, a muscarinic receptor antagonist with bladder selectivity and so fewer side-effects and increased compliance, is also available in long-acting XL form
    - anticholinergic agents are contraindicated in narrow angle glaucoma
    - topical oestrogens for urogenital atrophy may help relieve sensation of urgency.

2   Stress incontinence

- Second most common type of incontinence in elderly women.
- Urine leaks during physical activity, e.g. standing, lifting, coughing, sneezing, laughing (i.e. conditions of increased abdominal pressure).
- Weakness of pelvic floor and bladder neck lead to sphincter incompetence
- Causes include damage during childbirth and postmenopausal atrophy due to oestrogen deficiency.
- Men may develop post-prostatectomy stress incontinence due to iatrogenic sphincter damage.
- Treatment methods include:
  (i)   pelvic floor exercises:
     -   aim to improve tone of pelvic floor muscles especially levator ani
     -   vaginal examination essential to ensure ability to contract correct muscle before exercises are taught
     -   continence may take more than three months.
  (ii) biofeedback with a vaginal or rectal sensor can be used to monitor results of patient effort
  (iii) electrical stimulation helps pelvic floor develop new fibres
  (iv) hormone replacement therapy – urethra and trigone of bladder are sensitive to oestrogen
  (v)   surgery can be considered in some cases (comorbidity may preclude this).

3   Retention and overflow

- Large post-void residual volume.
- Continuous dribbling incontinence results.
- Recurrent urinary tract infections common.
- Constipation and anticholinergic drugs exacerbate symptoms.
- Causes include outflow tract obstruction, diabetes mellitus, injury to nerves supplying bladder.
- Detrusor underactivity unlikely to be the main problem.

4   Outflow obstruction

- Almost always in men.
- Symptoms include hesitancy, poor urinary stream, post-micturition dribbling and feeling of inadequate emptying.
- In chronic outflow obstruction detrusor may be replaced with fibrosis so bladder fails to empty even when obstruction is removed.
- Causes include benign prostatic hypertrophy (BPH), prostate cancer and urethral stricture.
- 1 in 3 men referred for prostatectomy because of obstructive symptoms have an overactive detrusor for which surgery is not appropriate.

- BPH:
  - (i)   prevalence rises with age (50% of men aged 50–60 and 90% of those aged over 85 years)
  - (ii) symptoms:
    - – irritative: urgency, frequency, nocturia, urge incontinence
    - – obstructive: hesitancy, straining, feeling of incomplete emptying, retention, overflow incontinence, poor stream
  - (iii) investigation: history, urinary symptoms review, rectal examination, urinalysis, renal function, PSA
  - (iv) refer to urologist if:
    - – moderate to severe symptoms
    - – history of recurrent urinary tract infections
    - – suspicious prostate
    - – PSA more than 4
    - – palpable bladder
    - – failure to respond to medical treatment
  - (v)   treatment depends on symptom severity and comorbidity
  - (vi) medical treatments:
    - – alpha-blockers, e.g. alfuzosin, doxazosin, tamsulosin
    - – 5 alpha-reductase inhibitors, e.g. finasteride
  - (vii) side-effects of TURP:
    - – 70% retrograde ejaculation
    - – 14% impotence
    - – urinary incontinence in up to 15%.

5   Functional

- Due to inability to reach and use toilet in time.
- Associated with poor mobility, loss of manual dexterity, confusion, communication problems and reduced motivation, e.g. depression.

6   Neurogenic

- Damage to neuronal control of bladder function.
- Different lesions cause different effects:
  - (i)   loss of voluntary inhibition causes frequency, urgency, incontinence (stroke, frontal lobe tumour)
  - (ii) atonic bladder leads to retention and overflow
  - (iii) spinal cord damage results in reflex voiding
  - (iv) local irritation, e.g. bladder stone or tumour causes sensory urgency +/− incontinence.

7   Mixed

- Combined urge and stress incontinence is common in older women.

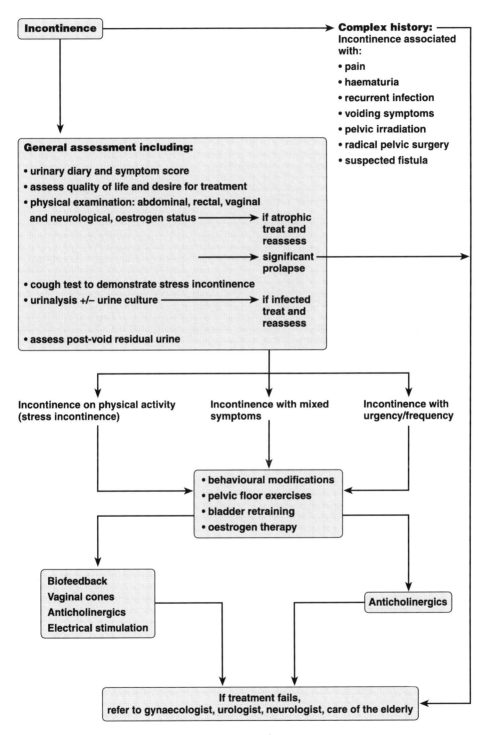

Figure 25.1   Incontinence treatment pathway.[1]

National Service Framework for Older People Standard 3: Patient-centred Care (2001)[2]

Integrated continence services

Aims

- To support older people and their carers.
- To be in line with published guidance on good practice.
- To link identification (community dwellers/care home residents/hospital inpatients), assessment and treatment across primary care and acute/specialist care.
- To provide links to designated specialties, e.g. urology and regional/national units for specialist surgery.
- To provide continence aids/equipment.
- To provide access to bathing and laundry services.

British Geriatrics Society: A Guide for Those Working in Residential and Nursing Homes (1998)[3]

Rationale

- Urinary incontinence should not be seen as inevitable.
- Many cases may be preventable.
- Good management should make untreatable cases more acceptable.

Assessment

- Establish patient's and carer's views of the problem and the impact it has on quality of life.
- Complete fluid balance and voiding charts.
- Ensure regular bowel action.

Management

- Ensure care home staff are trained in continence promotion.
- Provide assisted toileting for those with mobility/dexterity problems.
- Enlist assistance of GP to identify conditions that may exacerbate symptoms and treat as appropriate, e.g. infection, oestrogen deficiency, diabetes mellitus.
- Refer to continence nurse specialist for advice if required.
- Review medication and discontinue unnecessary drugs, e.g. diuretics, sedatives.
- Toileting regimes:
  - aim to ensure bladder emptying before incontinence occurs
  - optimum time between visits should be determined by voiding record.
- Continence pads:
  - available through community nursing or social services
  - various sizes and absorbencies
  - heavier pads for night-time use
  - mesh pants to keep in position
  - may lead to dependence and acceptance that incontinence is expected and irreversible.
- Sheaths:
  - need to ensure correct size
  - may cause local skin irritation and infection.
- Catheters:
  - intermittent catheterisation (self or staff) may be an option
  - long-term indwelling catheter may be required, e.g. persistent retention, non-healing pressure sores, to promote comfort
  - available on prescription
  - need to be changed every six weeks to prevent blockage
  - increase risk of infection
  - all have bacteriuria – only treat if symptomatic
  - may use leg bag or open valve at intervals.

Department of Health: Good Practice in Continence Services (2000)[4]

- Integrated services.
- Clinical audit.
- Identify conditions that may exacerbate incontinence, e.g. chronic cough.

- Staff training.
- General advice to patients and carers, e.g. diet/fluid intake.
- Bladder training.
- Pelvic floor and anal sphincter exercises.
- Review medication, e.g. diuretics.
- Manage faecal impaction.
- Measure changes in urinary symptoms from before treatment to six months later.
- Measure patient satisfaction six months after treatment.
- Issue continence aids only after an initial assessment and/or a management/treatment plan has been completed (prematurely can lead to psychological dependence and reluctance to attempt curative treatment).
- Improve staff knowledge about products, e.g. handheld urinals for women.

Other urinary complaints

Nocturia

- Greater than twice per night.
- Disrupts sleeping pattern.
- Older people pass more urine at night (redistribution of fluid, e.g. peripheral oedema, reduced renal concentrating ability and increased GFR in supine position).
- Careful timing of caffeine, alcohol and certain medications is required.

Polyuria

- Treat possible contributing causes, e.g. diabetes mellitus, hypercalcaemia, diabetes insipidus.

References

1 Abrahams P, Khoury S and Wein A (1999) Incontinence abstracts from Proceedings of the 1st International Consultation on Incontinence. Health Publications Ltd, London.
2 Department of Health (2001) *National Service Framework for Older People*. DoH, London.
3 British Geriatrics Society (1998) *Continence Care – A Guide for those Working in Residential and Nursing Homes*. Compendium Document B2.
4 Department of Health (2000) *Good Practice Incontinence Series*. DoH, London.

26

Gastro-oesophageal reflux disease

Definition

Gastro-oesophageal reflux disease is a backflow of gastric contents into the oesophagus resulting in oesophageal damage and/or a negative impact on quality of life as a result of dyspeptic symptoms.

Aetiology

- Prevalence of reflux-related symptoms rises with age (more than 20% of over-65s).
- Contributing factors include:
  - age-related changes in upper gastrointestinal tract
  - medication (especially NSAIDs)
  - difficulty maintaining an upright posture after eating.

Clinical features

- Heartburn (retrosternal/epigastric burning).
- Postprandial epigastric pain.
- Nocturnal symptoms may be associated with poor sleep and respiratory problems secondary to aspiration.
- Alarm features include:
  - dysphagia/odynophagia
  - persistent vomiting
  - unexplained weight loss
  - iron deficiency anaemia
  - abdominal mass.

Long-term consequences

- Barrett's oesophagus and oesophageal cancer.
- Oesophageal stricture/ulceration.
- Chronic cough.

Diagnosis

- May be complicated by:
  - atypical symptoms
  - comorbidity, e.g. ischaemic heart disease.
- Proton pump inhibitor (PPI) trial if no alarm features.
- British Society of Gastroenterology guidelines (1996) recommend endoscopy for patients with alarm features and those aged over 45 years (National Institute of Clinical Excellence (2000) suggests over 55 years).

Treatment

- General advice:
  - avoid large meals
  - avoid lying down after eating
  - lose weight if overweight
  - stop smoking
  - reduce alcohol intake
  - elevate head of bed.
- Discontinue contributing medication if possible (otherwise continue with PPI prophylaxis).
- PPIs are the treatment of choice.
- NICE guidelines for PPI use in dyspepsia:
  - Mild dyspepsia:
    (i) antacids, alginates or H2 receptor antagonists before PPI.
  - Severe dyspepsia:
    (i) healing dose PPI until symptoms controlled then lowest dose to maintain control
    (ii) restart at higher dose if recurrent symptoms.

27

Chronic obstructive pulmonary disease

Definition

- A disorder characterised by airflow obstruction, which is usually progressive, not fully reversible and does not change markedly over several months.
- Airflow obstruction is defined as a reduced FEV_1 (forced expiratory volume in 1 second) and a reduced FEV_1/FVC (forced vital capacity) ratio such that FEV_1 <80% predicted and FEV_1/FVC <0.7.
- Encompasses both chronic bronchitis and emphysema.

Pathology

- Chronic inflammation most commonly secondary to tobacco smoke leads to damage of the airways and lung parenchyma.

Statistics

- Results in 30 000 deaths in UK each year (sixth most common cause of death).
- A major cause of mortality and morbidity in older people.
- 1% of UK population have COPD (incidence rises steeply with age).
- Exerts considerable economic burden on NHS (£500 million/year).
- 12% of medical hospital admissions are for COPD.
- Average length of inpatient stay is 10 days.
- Responsible for majority of pressure during winter bed crises.

Diagnosis

- Underdetected and misdiagnosed.
- No single diagnostic test.

- Diagnosis should be based on a combination of:
  - spirometry (assessment of airway obstruction)
  - symptoms (shortness of breath, cough, reduced exercise capacity, fatigue, sleep disturbance, weight loss)
  - impact on quality of life (social/psychological morbidity).
- Exacerbations typically present with worsening dyspnoea, wheeze, chest tightness and productive cough (note change in sputum colour, consistency and volume).
- Early recognition of an exacerbation is vital.

Management

- Multidisciplinary approach to care.
- Smoking cessation should be encouraged at any age.
- Use of nicotine replacement products increases long-term abstinence.
- Short-acting inhaled bronchodilators are the mainstay of symptomatic treatment (beta2-agonist, e.g. salbutamol, or anticholinergic agent, e.g. ipratropium bromide).
- Long-acting inhaled bronchodilators (beta2-agonist, e.g. salmeterol, or anticholinergic, e.g. tiotropium) should be added if still symptomatic on short-acting preparations or if ≥ 2 exacerbations per year.
- Inhaled corticosteroids should be considered in patients with a FEV_1 $\leq 50\%$ predicted and who have had ≥ 2 exacerbations requiring treatment with antibiotics and/or oral steroids within 12 months.
- Ability to use an inhaler should be tested prior to initiating inhaled therapy and technique reviewed regularly.
- Spacer devices are available to ease administration of inhaled products.
- Nebulised bronchodilators will be required if disabling symptoms persist despite maximum inhaled treatment.
- Maintenance oral steroids may be required in advanced cases (remember osteoporosis prophylaxis).
- Theophyllines should only be prescribed after trials of short- and long-acting inhaled bronchodilators.
- Consider mucolytic agents in chronic productive cough.
- Long-term oxygen is indicated for patients with a pO2 <7.3 kPa when stable or 7.3–8 kPa when stable and one of the following is present: polycythaemia, nocturnal hypoxaemia, peripheral oedema or pulmonary hypertension.
- Offer annual influenza vaccination and pneumococcal vaccination.
- Consider antiviral agents (zanamivir, oseltamivir) for at-risk patients presenting within 48 hours of onset of influenza-like symptoms.

- Stress importance of responding promptly to symptoms of an exacerbation.
- NICE (2004)[1] recommends that patients who consider themselves to be functionally disabled by COPD should be offered pulmonary rehabilitation:
  - contraindications include immobility, unstable angina and recent myocardial infarction
  - programme should be tailored to individual needs
  - interventions include physical training, education, nutritional advice and assessment of psychological/social needs.
- Development of acute respiratory assessment services will place greater emphasis on community-based care, e.g. Hospital at Home for suitable patients, hence avoiding the emergency department.

Table 27.1 Factors to consider when deciding where to manage a patient with an exacerbation of COPD (NICE 2004)

Factor	Favours hospital treatment	Favours home treatment
Able to manage at home	No	Yes
Breathlessness	Severe	Mild
General condition	Poor/deteriorating	Good
Level of activity	Poor/confined to bed	Good
Cyanosis	Yes	No
Worsening peripheral oedema	Yes	No
Level of consciousness	Impaired	Normal
Already receiving LTOT	Yes	No
Social circumstances	Living alone/not coping	Good
Acute confusion	Yes	No
Rapid rate of onset	Yes	No
Significant comorbidity	Yes	No
SaO2 <90%	Yes	No
Chest x-ray changes	Yes	No
Arterial pH level	<7.35	$\geq$7.35
Arterial pO2	<7 kPa	$\geq$7 kPa

Reference

1 National Institute for Clinical Excellence (2004) *Management of Chronic Obstructive Pulmonary Disease in Primary and Secondary Care*. NICE, London.

28

Community-acquired pneumonia

Definition of pneumonia

- Symptoms and signs of an acute lower respiratory tract infection, including a cough and at least one other lower respiratory tract symptom, plus at least one systemic symptom, and new focal signs on chest examination.

Statistics

- A major cause of mortality and morbidity in older people.
- Responsible for 10% of all deaths in the UK each year.
- 70% of patients admitted to hospital with CAP are aged over 75.

Diagnosis

- Challenging in the older population.
- Clinical features may be atypical and non-specific, e.g. confusion.
- Fever may be absent.
- Microscopy and culture of sputum may yield the causative organism, but antibiotic treatment should not be delayed.
- Consider pulmonary tuberculosis if persistent productive cough, systemic symptoms or high-risk group (ethnic background, social deprivation).

Poor prognostic features

- British Thoracic Society (2001) 'CURB' score:[1]
  - **C**onfusion (new/mental test score <8)
  - **U**rea (>7)
  - **R**espiratory rate (>30/minute)
  - **B**lood pressure (systolic <90 mmHg +/or diastolic <60 mmHg)
  - ≥2 adverse features indicates a high risk of death.
- Other markers of poor prognosis:
  - age over 50 years
  - significant comorbidity, e.g. renal/heart failure
  - hypoxaemia (O2 saturations <90%/pO2 <8 kPa)
  - bilateral or multilobar involvement on chest film.

Management

- Most common organisms in elderly people are *Streptococcus pneumoniae*, *Haemophilus influenzae* and the influenza viruses.
- Chlamydia pneumonia may be important in residents of care homes.
- Place of management (home or hospital) depends on severity of episode.
- General measures include rest, smoking cessation, maintenance of hydration and simple analgesia for pleuritic chest pain.
- Early treatment with antibiotics in suitable patients shortens duration of illness and reduces mortality risk.
- BTS guidelines (2001) suggest amoxicillin 500 mg–1 g tds (or either erythromycin 500 mg qds or clarithromycin 500 mg bd if penicillin allergic) for at least a week.
- Patients (and/or carers) should be educated about when to seek help if managed at home – these cases require early medical review.

Reference

1 British Thoracic Society Guidelines on the management of community-acquired pneumonia. *Thorax*. **56** (Suppl. IV): 1–64.

29
Diabetes mellitus

Definition

Diabetes mellitus is a chronic, progressive disease characterised by a raised blood glucose level.

Pathology

- Type I: insulin insufficiency results from autoimmune destruction of insulin-secreting pancreatic beta-cells.
- Type II: results from defects in insulin secretion or insulin insensitivity.

Statistics

- Affects 1.3 million of the UK population (Type I 15%/Type II 85%).
- Incidence is increasing in all age groups (projected rise of more than 40% by 2023).
- One of the most common chronic diseases affecting elderly people.
- Prevalence rises with age (over 65 years: 1 in 20/over 85 years: 1 in 5).
- Most older people have Type II diabetes.
- More common in certain ethnic groups (South Asian, African, Afro-Caribbean and Middle Eastern).
- Diabetes care is costly – £4.9 billion/year (or 9% of total NHS budget).

Diagnosis

- Diabetes:
  - random plasma glucose >11.1 mmol/l
  - fasting plasma glucose >7 mmol/l
  - 2-hour post-prandial glucose >11.1 mmol/l

- Impaired glucose tolerance:
  - 2-hour post-glucose load 7.8–11.1 mmol/l
- Impaired fasting glucose:
  - fasting plasma glucose 6.1–6.9 mmol/l
- Normal:
  - fasting plasma glucose <6.1 mmol/l
  - 2-hour post-prandial glucose <7.8 mmol/l

Complications

- Life expectancy is reduced by more than 20 years in Type I and up to 10 years in Type II.
- Cardiovascular disease is the most common cause of death.
- Poor glycaemic control increases the risk of long-term consequences.
- United Kingdom Prospective Diabetes Study (UKPDS) 1998:[1] effective control of blood glucose and blood pressure can reduce/delay onset of complications.
- Microvascular complications:
  - retinopathy:
    (i) visual impairment
    (ii) blindness.
  - nephropathy – renal failure (microalbuminuria of more than 30 mg/l is an early indicator of renal involvement; proteinuria of more than 300 mg/day occurs in progressive disease).
  - neuropathy:
    (i) loss of sensation (predisposition to foot ulcers)
    (ii) postural hypotension
    (iii) impotence
    (iv) urinary retention
    (v) diarrhoea.
- Macrovascular complications:
  - cardiovascular:
    (i) ischaemic heart disease
    (ii) heart failure.
  - cerebrovascular:
    (i) stroke
    (ii) transient ischaemic attack.
  - peripheral – amputation.
- Other complications:
  - cataracts

- infections (skin/urine)
- loss of functional independence
- depression.

Treatment of Type II diabetes

- Dietary regulation.
- Increased physical activity.
- Patient/carer education.
- Control of hypertension and hyperlipidaemia.
- Smoking cessation.
- Secondary prevention measures for ischaemic heart disease (aspirin, beta-blockers).
- ACE inhibition for microalbuminuria.
- Regular foot care.
- Annual review (dilated eye examination, sensory testing, palpation of peripheral pulses).
- Individual care plan (home monitoring with district nurse support if required, realistic glycaemic goals).
- Oral treatment
  - Biguanides (e.g. metformin):
    (i) lower blood glucose primarily by reducing hepatic gluconeogenesis
    (ii) often used in overweight patients as weight loss may be a side-effect
    (iii) may cause lactic acidosis
    (iv) should be avoided in renal impairment
    (v) gastrointestinal side-effects such as anorexia and nausea may preclude use.
  - Sulphonylureas (e.g. gliclazide, glipizide):
    (i) increase pancreatic beta-cell secretion of insulin
    (ii) often used first line in non-overweight patients
    (iii) shorter-acting preparations preferred (avoid glibenclamide in view of long half-life).
  - Alpha-glucosidase inhibitors (e.g. acarbose):
    (i) inhibit conversion of non-absorbable starch and sucrose into absorbable monosaccharides such as glucose
    (ii) reduce rate of glucose uptake into bloodstream and lower post-prandial blood glucose levels
    (iii) modest effects only
    (iv) side-effects include abdominal bloating, flatulence and diarrhoea.

- Thiazolidinediones (e.g. pioglitazone, rosiglitazone):
  (i)   reduce peripheral and hepatic insulin resistance and decrease glucose levels by augmenting insulin-mediated peripheral glucose disposal
  (ii) used as a combination treatment in patients with insufficient glycaemic control despite maximum tolerated doses of either metformin or sulphonylurea
  (iii) avoid in cardiac/renal/hepatic failure.
- Metaglinides (e.g. repaglinide, nateglinide):
  (i)   stimulate release of insulin from pancreatic beta cells
  (ii) similar to sulphonylureas but act at separate sites
  (iii) short duration and fast action mean post-prandial glucose spikes are reduced
  (iv) can be used as monotherapy or with metformin
  (v)   avoid in hepatic impairment
  (vi) notable drug interactions: diuretics, ACE inhibitors, salicylates, alpha-blockers and statins.
- Insulin:
  (i)   required in Type I diabetes
  (ii) approximately 40% of patients with Type II diabetes will eventually need insulin
  (iii) indicated in Type II diabetes if poor glycaemic control with symptoms/persistently raised HbA1c > 9%/persistent ketonuria despite dietary regulation and maximal oral therapy, continuing weight loss, severe intercurrent illness, hyperosmolar non-ketotic coma (HONK) and in specific situations, e.g. post myocardial infarction
  (iv) aim is to simulate normal insulin secretion in response to dietary intake, exercise levels and metabolic state
  (v)   various regimens available (e.g. twice-daily regimen of a mixture of short and intermediate action insulin such as Human Mixtard 30/70 or once daily insulin glargine)
  (vi) pre-loaded pen devices simplify administration
  (vii) assistance of carers or district nurses may be required.

Home monitoring of glycaemic control

- Complicated by comorbidity, e.g. poor eyesight, arthritis, cognitive impairment.
- Urine dipstick monitoring pre-prandially once a week is often sufficient for patients with diet- or tablet-controlled Type II diabetes.

- Blood glucose monitoring is recommended for patients with Type I and those with Type II on insulin.
- Twice-daily BMs if poor control or four-point profile once weekly if stable.
- Fasting measurements of 7–9 mmol/l and random readings of 8–11 mmol/l should be sufficient to avoid hypo- and hyperglycaemic episodes.
- Tight control may not always be possible in older people:
  - risk of hypoglycaemia
  - intolerance of medication
  - polypharmacy/drug interactions.
- Hypoglycaemia:
  - predisposing factors include:
    (i) poor/erratic nutritional intake
    (ii) impaired perception or response to hypoglycaemia secondary to cognitive difficulties
    (iii) dependence or isolation limiting early treatment
    (iv) comorbidity leading to misdiagnosis
    (v) impaired renal/hepatic metabolism.
  - Glargine is a long-acting insulin analogue with more predictable glycaemic control. It is recommended by NICE for patients with frequent hypoglycaemic episodes, for those who require assistance from a carer or health professional to administer injections and for patients who would otherwise need twice-daily injections plus oral therapy.

Diabetes in care homes[2]

- 10% of care home residents have diabetes.
- A particularly vulnerable group.
- British Diabetic Association recommendations (1999):
  - screening on entry to care facility and then every two years
  - individualised diabetes care and dietary plans for all residents with known diabetes
  - support to enable residents to manage their diabetes where this is feasible
  - avoidance of unnecessary and inappropriate medical interventions
  - annual review (preferably in care home) including history, examination, review of glycaemic control and medication, dilated fundoscopy, assessment of visual acuity and renal function
  - access to health professionals including doctor, diabetes specialist nurse, dietician, podiatrist and optician
  - educational training programme for care home staff.

National Service Framework for Diabetes[3]

Relevant standards

- Prevention of Type II diabetes.
- Identification of people with diabetes.
- Empowering people with diabetes.
- Clinical care of adults with diabetes.
- Management of diabetic emergencies.
- Care of people with diabetes during admission to hospital.
- Detection and management of long-term complications.

References

1 UK Prospective Diabetes Study Group (1998) Tight blood pressure control and risk of macrovascular and microvascular complications in Type 2 Diabetes – UK PPS 38. *BMJ*. **317**: 703–13.
2 Guidelines and Practice for Residents with Diabetes in Care Homes (1999) A report prepared by a working party of the British Diabetic Association on behalf of the Diabetes Care Advisory Committee, London.
3 Department of Health (2001) *National Service Framework for Diabetes: National Standards*. DoH, London.

Part IV

Administrative aspects of services

30

Health and social services

Principles of good medical and social care for elders (British Geriatrics Society 2003)[1]

- Involvement of the older person in decisions on their future care.
- Promotion of good health.
- Prevention of illness.
- Reduction of disability.
- Provision of home support.
- Preservation of dignity, autonomy and respect.
- Elimination of age discrimination.

Acute medical care

Models of geriatric medicine

- Traditional – older adults with complex needs are admitted to the geriatric service.
- Age-defined – medical patients above a certain age are admitted under a geriatrician.
- Integrated – both elderly patients and younger adults are cared for by a general physician with an interest in geriatrics.
- No firm evidence is available to indicate which pattern of care provides the best outcome.

Aims

- Waiting time in the emergency department should be less than four hours before transfer or discharge.
- Inter-ward transfers should be minimal.
- Elderly patients admitted under a general medical team should see a geriatrician within 72 hours.
- Care should be delivered by an experienced multidisciplinary team skilled in dealing with the problems of old age.
- The need for rehabilitation should be identified as soon as possible.
- Discharge planning should commence early.
- Specialist opinions, investigations and treatment should not be compromised purely on the basis of age.

Specialist inpatient geriatric services

- Stroke – a specialist stroke service should be established in each trust.
- Orthogeriatrics – a pre- and post-operative care liaison service to include assessment of falls risk and bone protection should be available.
- General rehabilitation – either at the acute hospital site or other non-acute care facility.

Intermediate care

- A term that has been used in many different contexts.
- Born out of the National Beds Inquiry (2000), which emphasised the inappropriate use of many acute hospital beds.
- Aims to promote recovery and independence following acute inpatient care provision or as an alternative to acute medical admission.
- Encompasses a range of services including:
  - rapid response
  - supported discharge
  - inpatient rehabilitation
  - hospital at home
  - day rehabilitation.
- Is the focus of Standard Three of the National Service Framework for Older People.

Rehabilitation

- An active process by which those people who are disabled by injury or disease achieve a full recovery or realise their optimal physical, mental and social potential and are integrated into their most appropriate environment (World Health Organization).
- Recovery from illness often takes longer in older people.
- Rehabilitation is an essential component of geriatric practice.
- Success relies on a multidisciplinary approach with effective communication between members of the team.
- Focus can be general or specific, e.g. stroke or orthogeriatric rehabilitation.
- Care can be provided in the inpatient setting or may be community based.
- Stages of the rehabilitation process (British Geriatrics Society 1997):[2]
  - Assessment – identification of problems
  - Planning – analysis of problems and goal setting
  - Treatment – intervention to reduce disability and handicap
  - Evaluation – assessment of effectiveness of intervention
  - Care – alleviation of any consequences of disability
  - Advice – development of coping strategies for patients and carers.

Continuing care

- NHS-funded hospital-based care for patients who have particularly difficult continuing medical, physical, psychological and emotional needs and in whom there is no potential for improvement.
- Rapid expansion in private care capacity over the last three decades means that nursing home places now outnumber continuing care beds by 2:1.
- Eligibility criteria for entry to continuing care facilities vary between health authorities – nationally agreed policies should be implemented.

Respite care

- Can be provided in the NHS or social service facilities depending on the patient's requirements.
- May be an isolated episode or part of a programme to relieve carer stress
- A good opportunity to reassess the needs of both patients and carers.

Outpatient clinical care

- A means of seeking a non-urgent geriatric medical assessment.
- Clinics may be general or specialized, e.g. falls, memory, continence.
- Access to multidisciplinary advice/input should be available.
- Smooth running depends on reliable transport services for disabled patients.
- Long waiting times should be avoided.

Geriatric day hospitals

- Originally developed in the UK in the 1960s.
- Benefits have been controversial for many years.
- May avoid admission to hospital or institutional care.
- Act as an interface between hospital and community services.
- Services provided include functional assessment, medical review and treatment if required and rehabilitation if appropriate.
- Patients attend for half/full days depending on need.
- Roles may extend to information provision, health education, respite for carers and opportunity for social interaction.

NHS community services

Services include:

- district nursing
- physiotherapy
- occupational therapy
- continence advice
- speech and language therapy
- dietetics
- podiatry.

Domiciliary visits

- A visit to a patient's home by a specialist, normally a consultant, at the request of the GP and normally in his or her company, to advise on the diagnosis or treatment of a patient who, on medical grounds, cannot attend the hospital (Department of Health and Social Services 1981).

- In reality joint visits rarely occur.
- Advantages:
  - may avoid inappropriate admissions
  - provide valuable information about the home circumstances.
- Criticisms:
  - time consuming
  - abuse of the system through inappropriate referrals.

Psychogeriatric services

- Specialist mental health services for the elderly have expanded over recent years.
- Services include:
  - psychogeriatric inpatient care
  - old age psychiatry and care of the elderly inpatient liaison
  - outpatient clinics including specialised services, e.g. memory
  - long-stay institutional care (NHS and private facilities)
  - community-based assessment and treatment
  - domiciliary visits
  - outreach visits to nursing and residential homes.

Social services

- Social care encompasses a wide range of services provided by local authorities and the private sector including home care assistance, meals on wheels, day centres and residential/nursing home facilities.
- The Care Standards Act (2000) was developed as part of the government's plan to modernise social care by regulating all social care services including care homes in accordance with national minimum standards.

Long-term placement

- If a patient is unable to return home after treatment and rehabilitation, they may expect to receive care in another setting depending on their needs.
- Alternative types of accommodation include sheltered housing, residential care, nursing home care or long-stay wards in hospital.

Care homes

- Elderly people in care homes can be very vulnerable.
- The Royal College of Physicians has established a set of guidelines designed to optimise their care:[3]
  - a standardised interdisciplinary approach to assessment, care planning and care delivery should be adopted
  - all practitioners engaged in care home services should have appropriate training
  - a geriatrics nurse specialist and GP with a special interest in care of the elderly should play key roles
  - consultant outreach sessions would be useful.

References

1 British Geriatrics Society (1997) *Standards of Medical Care for Older People: Expectations and recommendations*. Compendium Document A3. Revised January 2003. British Geriatrics Society, London.
2 British Geriatrics Society (1997) *Rehabilitation of Older People*. Compendium Document A4. British Geriatrics Society, London.
3 Royal College of Physicians Working Party Report (2000) *The Health and Care of Older People in Care Homes*. RCP, London.

31

Income maintenance

Pensions

State pension

- The amount of basic state pension one receives depends upon the qualifying years one has built up before reaching state pension age (60 for females and 65 for males).
- A man will receive the full state pension if he has 44 years of qualifying years.
- The full basic pension is £79.60 a week for a single person and £127.25 for a couple.
- For a female, 39 qualifying years are required in order to get the full basic pension – this rule applies before 2010.
- When the pension age for women and men becomes 65, the number of qualifying years a woman needs to get the full state pension will increase to 44 years.
- People who do not qualify for the full basic state pension but who have more than 25 per cent of qualifying years will get a basic state pension between the minimum (£19.36 a week in 2003/04) and maximum (£79.60 a week in 2003/04).
- For those aged 80 years who do not have a state pension, there is a non-contributory state pension provided the person lives in the UK, has lived in the UK for a total of 10 years or more in any continuous period of 20 years after their 60th birthday and has no basic state pension, or less than 60% of the full rate.

Pension credit

Pension credit guarantees that everyone aged 60 and over has an income of at least:

- £105.10 per week for a single person
- £160.95 per week for a couple.

It will also reward people aged 65 and over for saving. For those who have saved they may get up to:

- £14.79 a week if single
- £19.20 a week for couples.

Annuities

- An annuity by definition is an exchange of a pension lump sum in return for an income from an insurance company.
- Once the annuity has been purchased a person cannot ever get the lump sum back.
- An annuity can be purchased any time between the ages of 50 and 75. The annuity rates depend upon the person's life expectancy, the amount in the pension fund and the economic conditions at the time of purchase.
- Compulsory purchase annuities relate to pension funds and the rules state that a person must purchase an annuity with his/her pension fund (net of any tax-free cash entitlement) by a maximum age of 75.
- Proposals to extend this age have been laid down by the government, but these new rules are not expected to become effective until at least April 2005.
- Purchased life annuities relate to non-pension monies and allow someone with a lump sum of capital to convert that to a regular income for life if they wish.
- Basic conventional annuities have a number of different options.

Level annuities – fixed level annuities

- These pay a guaranteed fixed level of income for life.
- Disadvantage of a level annuity – it provides no insurance against inflation and it allows the annuitant's income to fall steadily further behind average incomes if there is economic growth. For this reason potential annuitants might be better advised to purchase index-linked or escalating annuities.

Escalating annuities

- Payment increases every year, although initially the income will start at a lower level and will take a number of years before it reaches the amount available from a level annuity.

Spouse's pension

- This option allows someone to ensure that their spouse will continue to enjoy an income (typically 50%) after their death. Again this will usually mean a lower starting pension because of the probability that the annuity provider will be paying out for longer.

Guaranteed period

- This allows a person to have their pension paid for a guaranteed minimum period even if they die during this period. Typically the options are either five or 10 years.

There are also other types of annuities.

Section 32 annuities

- Also known as section 32 buyouts
- Allow people to transfer company pension scheme benefits to a private fund.

Income drawdown

- Allows a person to draw any tax-free cash entitlement and then draw an income between government set guidelines, which can be varied depending on your requirements.

Impaired annuities/enhanced annuities

- Allow higher annuity rates if an individual is suffering or has suffered from a number of medical conditions that could shorten life expectancy, e.g. high-blood pressure, cancer, strokes, heart attacks, etc.

Immediate annuities

- Enable a person to draw income from their pension fund now rather than at a future date.

Purchase life annuities

- These allow one to purchase an annuity from funds that did not originate from a pension fund, i.e. non-pension savings. They work in much the same way as an annuity from a pension, but with one notable and extremely beneficial difference.
- Under pension rules the annuity a person receives from a pension fund is treated as taxable income in the same way as income from normal employment would be. However, if a person uses other monies to buy a purchased life annuity, the tax treatment is different.
- Some of the income received is treated as capital, which is not taxed, and therefore the tax burden is reduced. The example below (based on a 65-year-old male, basic rate taxpayer with £100 000) illustrates the point:

  1 Pension annuity – Gross income = £7370, tax = £1621, net income = £5749
  2 Purchased life annuity – Gross income = £7370, tax = £367, net income = £7003.

- The illustration assumes that both annuities have the same gross income payable.

Care fee annuities

- These new annuities aim to provide a guaranteed income in return for a lump sum to pay for care in a residential or nursing home.

Other benefits/allowances available for older people

Winter fuel payment

- £200.00 for those aged 60 and over
- £300.00 for those aged 80 or over.

Housing benefit (rent allowance/rent rebate)

- This help towards rent is paid by local councils – the maximum available is the eligible rent.
- To obtain this a person does not need to get any other benefit.
- It does not cover mortgage interest.
- Can be claimed up to 13 weeks before one becomes entitled to it.

Housing benefit is determined by:

- savings a person and their partner have
- money that is coming in the form of earnings, some benefits, occupational pension and tax credit.

The other factors that will be taken into account by the local council are:

- the amount of rent for the particular home
- the home is a reasonable size for the person and their family
- the area the home is in.

The Appeals Decision made by the council can be challenged and appeal made to an independent appeal tribunal administered by the Appeal Service.

Attendance allowance (AA)

This benefit is paid if a person becomes ill or disabled on or after their 65th birthday. The rate of payment is dependent upon the care needs during the day, during the night or both. The AA can be claimed even if no one is actually giving the care. It is not affected by savings or other money an older person is getting.

The amount paid is:

- higher rate £57.20 per week
- lower rate £38.30 per week.

Payment of AA usually stops four weeks after an individual goes into a residential care or nursing home and this is arranged by social services. If the move is arranged by an individual and they are paying for the care, then they can continue to receive the AA.

Carer's allowance (CA)

Paid to full-time carers aged 16 and over who are spending at least 35 hours a week looking after someone who is getting:

- Attendance Allowance.
- Disability Living Allowance at the middle or highest rate for personal care.
- Industrial Injuries Disablement Benefit Constant Attendance Allowance.
- War Pensions Constant Attendance Allowance.

However, the carer cannot get the CA if they are in full-time education or earning above a certain amount.

Carer's allowance is currently (2004) £44.35.

Further information

www.pensions.gov.uk
www.thepensionservice.gov.uk
Citizens Advice – www.nacab.org.uk
www.info4pensioners.org.uk
www.dwp.gov.uk/lifeevent/benefits/housing_benefit.asp

32

Audit principles

Audit is defined as the systematic critical analysis of the quality of clinical care, including procedures used for diagnosis and treatment, the use of resources, the resulting outcome and quality of life for the patient. The purpose of audit should be educational and relevant to patient care.

To perform a successful audit cycle, a systematic approach is essential involving the stages outlined in Figure 32.1.

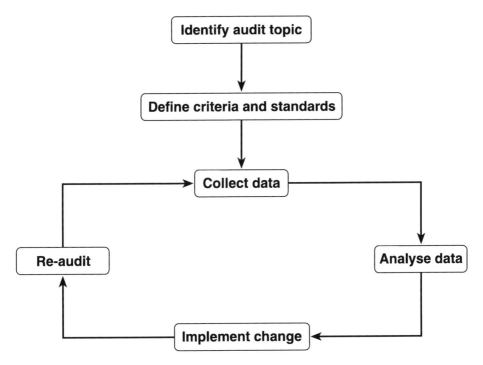

Figure 32.1 The audit cycle.

There are several approaches to clinical audit including:

- sentinel case audit, which examines variations from the norm in terms of outcome
- random case note review, which examines standards of note-keeping and quality of administrative documentation
- criterion-based review, which examines departures from specified criteria
- outcome review
- patient satisfaction, which aims to improve service delivery.

Audit standards in the elderly

- Need to reflect the special nature of healthcare of older people (atypical presentation, multiple pathologies, functional impairment and need for multidisciplinary assessment and treatment).
- Need to take account of national policy (NSF), good practice recommendations (NICE), as well as local professional and service experience in establishing principles.
- Standards need to be measurable, reflect success or failure of outcome and be locally determined on a multidisciplinary basis.
- The standards set should cover:
  - service organisation
  - service delivery
  - service evaluation
  - training, education and research and reflect the needs of the local population and not just the service.

Further reading

Dickinson E and Sinclair AJ (1989) Clinical audit of health care. In: MSJ Pathy (ed) *Principles and Practice of Geriatric Medicine*. John Wiley & Sons, Chichester.

Index